Experience Is the Best Teacher

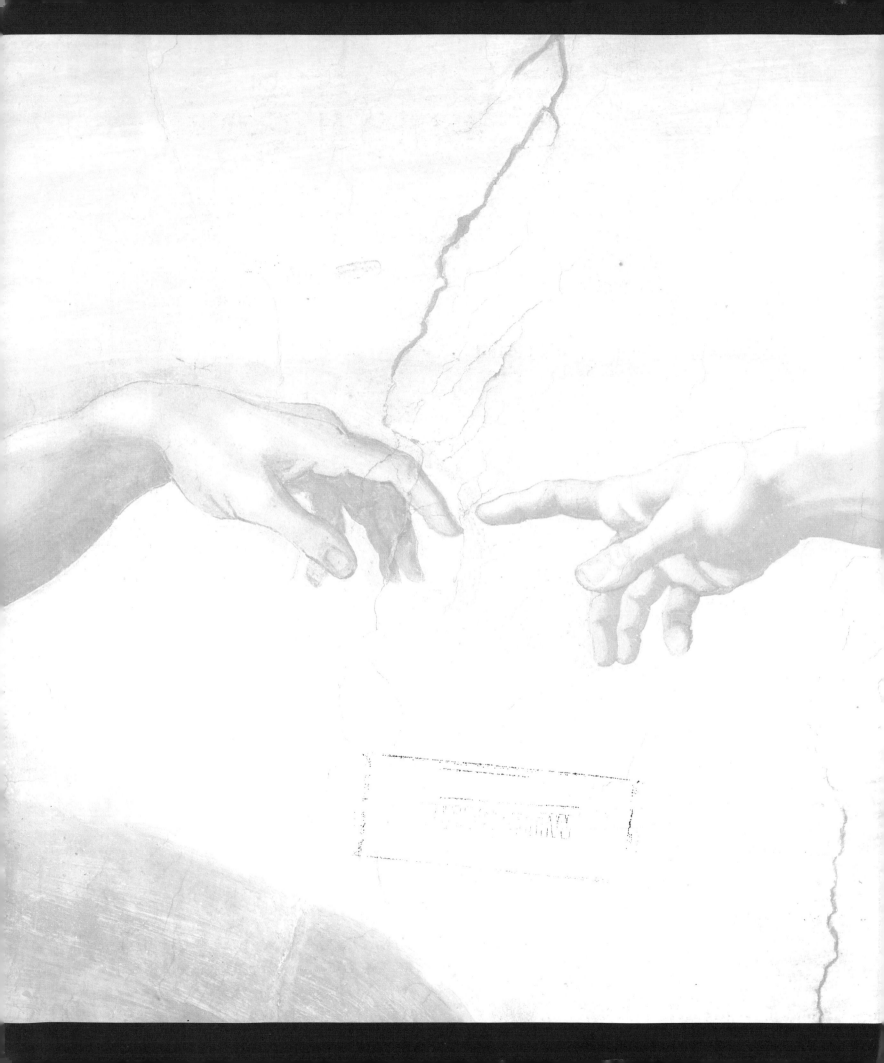

MANUAL OF DENTAL HYGIENE

EXPERIENCE
IS THE BEST TEACHER

Antonella Tani Botticelli

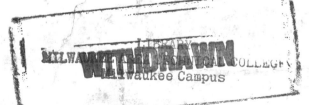

Quintessence Publishing Co, Inc
London, Chicago, Berlin, Tokyo, Paris, Barcelona, São Paulo,
New Delhi, Moscow, Prague, Warsaw, and Istanbul

quintessence
books

Botticelli, Antonella Tani
    Experience is the best teacher: manual of dental hygiene
    1. Dental hygiene - Handbooks, manuals, etc.
    I. Title
    617.6'01

ISBN 1-85097-047-5

Published by Quintessence Publishing Co, Inc
Grafton Road, New Malden
Surrey, KT3 3AB, UK

First published as *L'esperienza è la migliore insegnante: Manuale di igiene dentale,*
Antonella Tani Botticelli in Italian in 1999 by Ariminum Odontolgica srl, Rimini, Italy.

Clinical photographs: Daniele Botticelli, MD; Antonio Renzi, MD; and Antonella Tani Botticelli, DH
Prosthodontic reconstruction: Orthodontic Laboratory Secchiaroli A. and Carloni F., Rimini, Italy
Illustrations (marked DB): Daniele Botticelli, MD
Cover and page design: AMP, Rimini, Italy
Cover: Michelangelo (1475–1564), "The Creation of Adam," The Sistine Chapel, Vatican. Reprinted
with permission from SCALA Istituto Fotografico Editoriale Spa, Florence, Italy.

Printed in Germany

To my husband Daniele and our son Davide

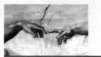

FOREWORD

This is not a traditional textbook of dental hygiene. It is a manual of dental hygiene.

It is a book written in a unique manner by a unique person, Antonella Tani Botticelli. It is a book created by a person with in-depth knowledge of the field of periodontology and dental hygiene, including both theoretic and practical aspects of the profession. Experience is the best teacher.

It is a book written by a dedicated dental hygienist for whom the well-being of her patients is ceaselessly in focus. In all the various chapters of this text, you will find information applicable for your work in the clinic. The information is delivered in an attractive, personal style and is easy to understand and utilize.

The book is intended for the student of dental hygiene, but may very well also serve as a manual for the student of dentistry as well as the practicing doctor of dental medicine.

It is with great pride and with much appreciation that I compliment Antonella for her achievements.

Jan T. Lindhe, LDS, Dr Odont, DMD
Professor and Chairman
Department of Periodontology
Göteborg University
Sweden

Dental hygienists are indispensable coworkers in modern dental offices that provide prophylactic services. They are also important in the practices of periodontists and dentists treating various degrees of periodontal diseases. To invest in the education of dental hygienists is therefore a fruitful and promising enterprise. To date, there are not too many textbooks written for dental hygienists. Instead, dental hygiene students have to study using textbooks and manuals written for their professional colleagues.

This new book is written for the dental hygienist and by a dental hygienist, Antonella Tani Botticelli. The author draws on numerous years of clinical involvement both with patients and with dental education. She is an enthusiastic and committed person whose practical courses throughout the years have been appreciated by many dental hygiene colleagues and professionals. Antonella Tani Botticelli has an unusual didactic feeling for the relevant clinical aspects of the profession. She masters the fields of periodontology, prevention, and patient handling extremely well. It doesn't come as a surprise, therefore, that her manual of dental hygiene sets the correct priorities and provides all the necessary information both for dental hygiene students as well as for those who would like to complete or refresh their understanding of the field. The practicing dentist may also profit from this unique manual. It can be recommended to all those who continuously strive for improvement in our profession. I congratulate Antonella Tani Botticelli for creating such a unique and down-to-earth book. Indeed, "experience is the best teacher."

Niklaus P. Lang, Dr Med Dent, MS, PhD, FRCPS (Glasg)
Professor and Chairman
Department of Periodontology and Fixed Prosthodontics
University of Berne
Switzerland

PREFACE

This book is intended for the student of dental hygiene, but those who already work in the profession may also find it useful. The text describes some important aspects of the work of a dental hygienist, and it is based on the experience accumulated during my 10 years in the profession.

The manual is divided into seven chapters—Periodontal Therapy, Motivation, Plaque Control at Teeth and Implants, Scaling and Root Planing, Instrument Sharpening, Treatment of Dental Hypersensivity, and Maintenance Therapy at Teeth and Implants—that deal with various aspects of periodontal therapy.

The successful treatment of periodontal disease is dependent on a close cooperation between skilled professionals (dental hygienists and dentists) and the patient. After a careful examination of the patient with periodontal disease, the dentist must choose the appropriate periodontal therapy and organize an adequate treatment plan. Many scientific publications and textbooks related to periodontology affirm that the patient has to receive detailed information about periodontal disease and the relationship between its emergence and progression and the presence of dental plaque. The patient must, that is, be correctly informed if they are then to be adequately motivated.

However, few attempts have been made to describe how such detailed information may be presented and which problems must be overcome in order to make the patient properly motivated for the treatment intended. One aspect of the problem is related to describing the disease to the patient. The professional often uses a technical medical language to describe the etiology and treatment of periodontal disease, instead of choosing words that are easy for the patient to understand. During my work as a dental hygienist, I have encountered many different types of patients, and years of experience have taught me how to communicate and establish a successful collaboration with those who arrive at the dental office initially unaware of what periodontal disease means. In this book, I offer the reader practical advice regarding various aspects of the process of motivation, and I indicate some examples that can be used to help people affected with periodontitis to understand their disease more easily.

Once patients have been thoroughly informed about their problem and decide to take measures to resolve it, the task of the hygienist is to teach the correct procedures to be used in the home care of teeth and/or implants. An ample portion of this text therefore deals with oral hygiene and the various instruments that may be recommended to help the patient achieve satisfactory results in a self-performed oral hygiene program. Practical suggestions are also offered on how to choose the proper toothbrush, brushing technique, appropriate interdental instruments, and other adjunctive devices that may be necessary.

Professional cleaning must, however, be performed when home care alone is not sufficient to resolve the patient's problem. In order to achieve adequate results, the hygienist must possess not only technical skill, but also good knowledge of the instruments used in periodontal treatment. Therefore, the fundamental characteristics of instruments for scaling are explained in a specific chapter that indicates with particular attention those that have enabled me to achieve excellent results even in cases where deep periodontal pockets were present. In the same section of the text, I also offer suggestions that I believe will be useful not only for operators who are right-handed, but also for those who are left-handed or ambidextrous.

The sharpening of instruments is another important aspect of the hygienist's role. Maintaining unchanged the initial characteristics of curettes has always been a big problem, but it can be resolved using an extremely simple method of sharpening that is explained in detail.

During or immediately after the active phase of periodontal treatment, the patient may complain of dental hypersensitivity. This problem may be alleviated or solved, and the various methods that I have learned to prefer and have found to be effective are described in a chapter of this text.

Once the active phase of treatment has been completed, maintenance therapy must follow in order to avoid recurrence of the disease. The chapter related to this aspect of periodontal treatment offers practical advice as to what should be done during a recall oral hygiene appointment and the way in which an efficient hygiene service should be organized.

In writing this book, I have tried to use a direct, cordial style of communication, and I have also chosen to omit captions near the pictures in order to integrate the photographic documentation and drawings directly into the text to render its reading more fluid. I hope readers will find this manual both easy to consult and helpful in improving or refreshing their knowledge of some of the essential aspects of dental hygiene.

Antonella Tani Botticelli

Antonella Tani Botticelli

ACKNOWLEDGMENTS

Special thanks to my husband Daniele for seeing in me qualities that I did not realize I had, for constantly supplying me with practical and psychological support, for conveying his tenacity to me, and for insisting that I obtain my diploma as a dental hygienist at a moment in which I thought it would be impossible to reconcile my family with my studies.

Sincere thanks to Prof Jan Lindhe and Prof Niklaus P. Lang for everything they have taught me, their indispensable advice, and for expressing their esteem for me, as a hygienist and as a person, in the forewords of this book.

Thanks also to Irene Riccitelli Guarella, DH, who was the first person to help me understand the real meaning of the word "motivation," and who also encouraged me to finish my studies.

Finally, I wish to thank all the assistants in the dental office where I work for helping me to prepare the photographs that accompany the text, and I also express my gratitude to all those who in some other way have contributed to the realization of this book.

CONTENTS

CONTENTS

CONTENTS

► **Chapter 7**

MAINTENANCE THERAPY AT TEETH AND IMPLANTS   181

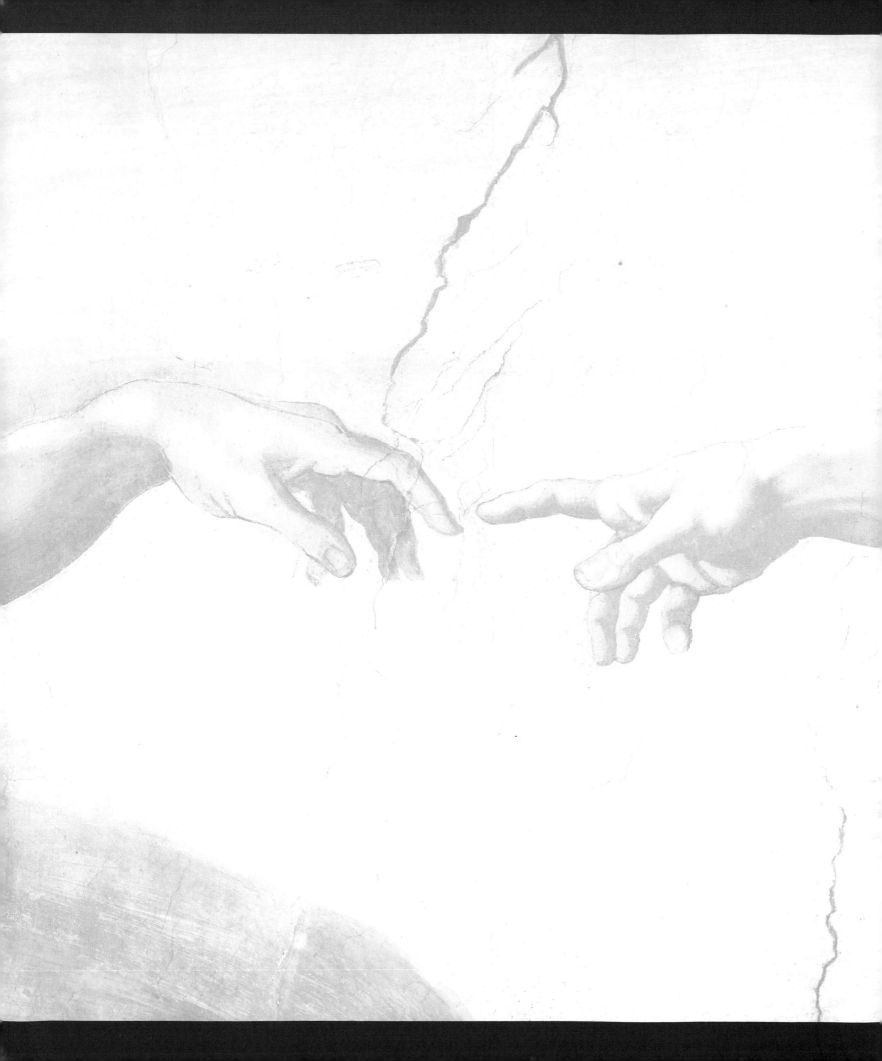

EXPERIENCE
IS THE BEST TEACHER

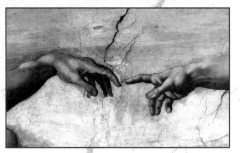

CHAPTER 1

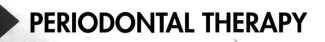

▶ PERIODONTAL THERAPY

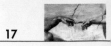
▶ EXAMINATION OF A PATIENT AFFECTED BY PERIODONTAL DISEASE

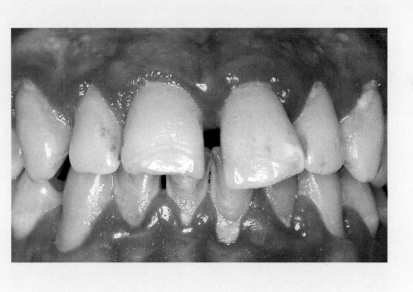

Bacterial plaque is the etiologic agent of periodontal disease[20,21]; this pathology neither emerges nor progresses in its absence. In order to formulate a specific treatment plan, a dentist must recognize the various types of periodontal lesions when conducting a careful examination of the patient's status.

Clinically, periodontitis is characterized both by alterations in the color and form of the gingiva, which becomes red and swollen, and by an increased tendency to bleed during probing in the sulcus or pocket.[19] Moreover, the periodontal tissue may present tissue recession and/or less resistance to probing, and the advanced phases of the disease are frequently associated with increased tooth mobility and migration of teeth. Loss of alveolar bone is verified through radiographic analysis.

In order to assess the quantity of supporting tissue that has been lost due to periodontal disease and identify the apical extension of the inflammatory lesion, the periodontal conditions of the buccal, lingual, and interproximal surfaces of all teeth must be examined and the following parameters entered in the patient's clinical chart:

- **Probing depth**
- **Bleeding on probing**
- **Probing attachment level**
- **Furcation involvement**
- **Tooth mobility**
- **Oral hygiene**

The dentist gathers these data during the patient's initial sitting. They are then reevaluated after the active treatment and subsequently during maintenance therapy.

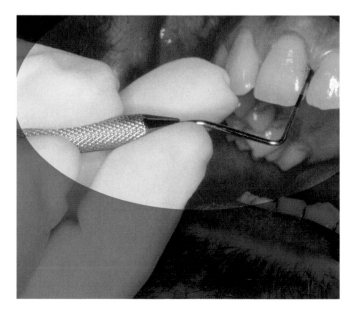

▷ **PROBING DEPTH**

The apical extent of the gingival lesion can be assessed by measuring the depth of the pocket.

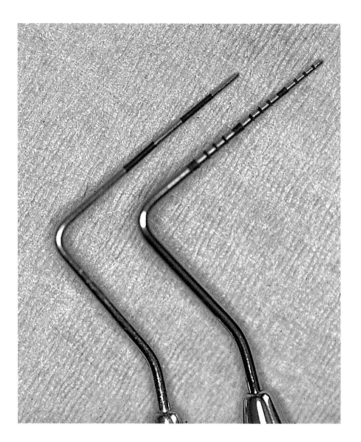

The instrument used for this measurement is the periodontal probe (eg, CP12 Williams, Hu-Friedy, Chicago, IL). This instrument is composed of a handle, a shank, and a thin working part that must have a blunt tip, a round cross section, and an easily readable millimeter scale.

The probe is used with a modified pen grasp: the tip of the middle finger is placed on the point of junction between the shank and the handle, and the thumb and the index finger hold the rest of the instrument; the ring finger is used as support, resting on the teeth as near as possible to the site of instrumentation.

Probing is effected by delicately inserting the probe, with a very light grasp, until it reaches the bottom of the sulcus or pocket, keeping the working part of the instrument parallel to the surface of the tooth.

A soft, elastic resistance will indicate that the base of the pocket or sulcus has been reached. The probing depth is the distance from the gingival margin to the deepest part of the pocket. The reading on the graduated probe is taken, and the measurement is scored on the patient's clinical chart.

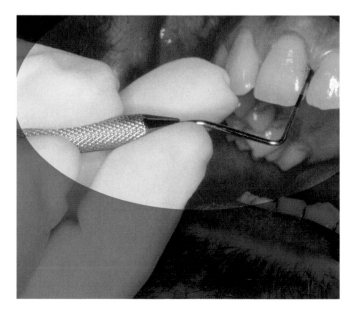

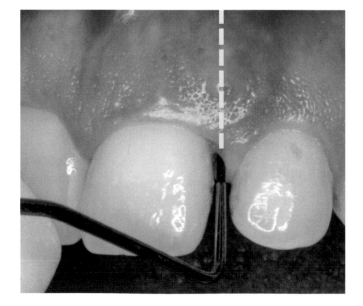

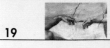
The probe is used with an uninterrupted, smooth, gentle up-and-down movement along the root surface of the tooth, and care is taken not to withdraw the instrument from the gingival margin at every movement.

The depth of the pockets is measured on all buccal, lingual and/or palatal, distal, and mesial surfaces. It is sufficient to score the deepest measurement of each of the four sides. Pockets that are < 4 mm may be excluded since they are not considered pathologic.

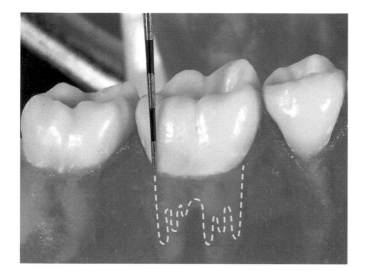

INITIAL EXAMINATION — B. Maria 38

Tooth	PROBING DEPTH 04/06/93				Furc Inv	Mob	Tooth	PROBING DEPTH				Furc Inv	Mob
	m	b	d	l				m	b	d	l		
18							48	4*					1
17	5*	5*	9*		D1	3	47	6*		4*	4	L1	1
16	5*		5*		D1		46	5*	4	6*			
15	5*	4	5*	4*		2	45	5*		4*			1
14	5*		5*	4		2	44						
13	5*		5*			1	43	5*					
12	6*		5*	4		1	42	4*		4*	4*		1
11	6*		6*	5*		1	41	4*					
21	6*		6*	4*		1	31	5*		5*	4*		2
22	5*		5*	6*		1	32	5*	4*	5*	4*		1
23	4*	5*	5*			1	33	5*		5*			
24			4*			1	34	5*		4*			1
25	5*					1	35			4*			
26	5*		6*			1	36	5*		5*			
27	6*	5*	6*			1	37	5*		6*		B1, L1	1
28	5*						38	6*		5*	6*		1

▷ BLEEDING ON PROBING

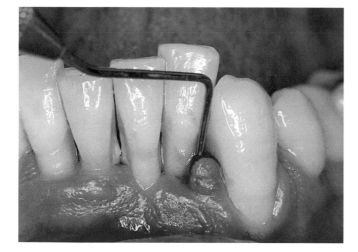

If the periodontal probe is inserted to the bottom of the gingival pocket and such instrumentation provokes bleeding, this signifies that there is inflammatory cell infiltrate and subgingival plaque in the area probed. This clinical sign is an important indicator of disease, and it is charted with an asterisk (*) beside the measurement of the pocket.

A correct choice of the periodontal probe and a careful exam procedure help to reduce or avoid errors of measurement that may depend on factors such as the diameter of the probe used, the variations in the probing force applied on the instrument during probing, the degree of inflammation in the tissues, an improper angulation of the probe, and/or the presence of pseudopockets and calculus.

Although these factors may be present, probing is still an effective means that can be used to evaluate periodontal tissue, above all when the information obtained is related to other findings such as bleeding on probing and variations in height of the alveolar bone assessed by means of the radiographic status.

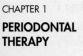
▷ **PROBING ATTACHMENT LEVEL**

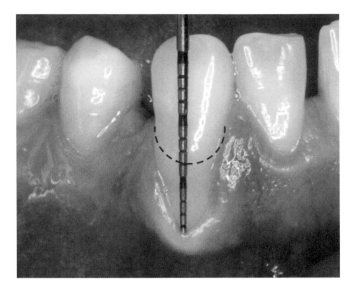

Attachment levels may be assessed with the use of a Williams periodontal probe and expressed in millimeters measuring the distance from the cementoenamel junction to the bottom of the gingival pocket. Today, few clinicians take these measurements because they are time-consuming and have little significance; what is really important is the amount of residual periodontal tissue, which is principally assessed by means of radiographic examination. However, probing of attachment level is indicated when the patient presents a degree of gingival recession that requires control during maintenance therapy.

The greatest distance for each surface concerned is recorded in the periodontal chart.

▷ **FURCATION INVOLVEMENT**

The destructive process of periodontal disease around multirooted teeth may involve the supporting structures of the furcation area. The Nabers No. 2 (Hu-Friedy) probe is used to identify the presence and extent of this destructive process.

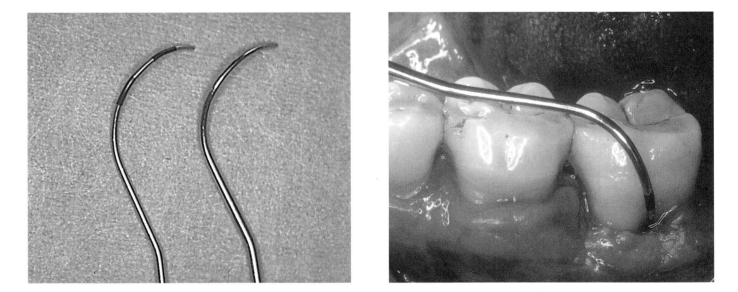

Furcation involvement may be classified by taking a horizontal measurement:

Degree I: Furcation can be probed to a depth that corresponds to one third of the width of the tooth.

Degree II: Furcation can be probed to a depth exceeding one third of the width of the tooth, but not through the total width.

Degree III: Furcation can be probed through the entire width of the furcation area.

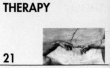

▷ TOOTH MOBILITY

Even though it is not the only cause, the continuous loss of supporting tissues in the progression of periodontal disease may result in increased tooth mobility.

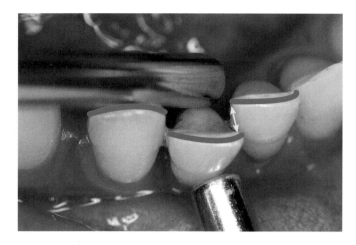

This increase in mobility may be classified as:

Degree I: Mobility of the crown of the tooth 0.2 to 1 mm in the horizontal direction

Degree II: Mobility of the crown of the tooth that exceeds 1 mm in the horizontal direction

Degree III: Mobility of the crown of the tooth in the vertical direction as well

▷ ORAL HYGIENE

The patient's oral hygiene must also be evaluated through the examination of the periodontal tissue. Alterations of the gingiva and the presence of bacterial plaque may be evidenced by means of indices.

In the clinical chart, each tooth is represented by a square and each tooth surface by a triangle:

• The upper triangle represents the buccogingival unit.
• The lower triangle represents the linguopalatal gingival unit.
• The two remaining triangles represent the interproximal gingival units.

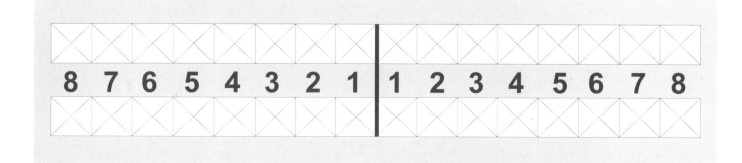

Each triangle that corresponds to a tooth surface where bleeding or plaque is present is colored. The mean value is expressed as a percentage.

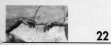
GINGIVAL BLEEDING INDEX[1]

The probe is moved gently along the marginal portion of the sulcus or the pocket and, after a pause of about 10 seconds, the results are observed.

The degree of gingivitis may be assessed when the clinical chart is compiled. Separate recordings are made, corresponding to the four surfaces of each tooth: the presence of bleeding is indicated by a colored triangle, and the absence of bleeding is indicated by a white triangle.

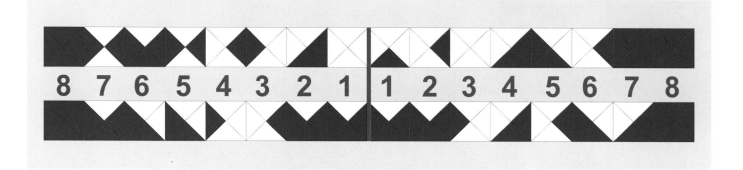

The Gingival Bleeding Index can be calculated once these scores have been completed:

$$\frac{67 \text{ (number of areas with bleeding)}}{128 \text{ (number of areas examined)}} \times 100 = 52.3 \text{ \%}$$

This index expresses the precise extent of gingivitis. It may also be called the "cooperation index" because it evidences the correct information regarding the patient's collaboration.

In the presence of plaque, a high Gingival Bleeding Index indicates that plaque has been accumulating long enough to provoke inflammation. In the absence of plaque, a high gingival bleeding index indicates that the plaque had been removed by the patient just a short while before his dental appointment and, therefore, there was not enough time for the inflammation to subside.

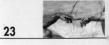
PLAQUE INDEX[30]

The presence of plaque can be detected by staining it with a disclosing solution.

The degree of plaque control may be assessed when the clinical chart is compiled. Separate recordings are made corresponding to the four surfaces of each tooth: the presence of plaque is indicated by a colored triangle, and the absence of plaque is indicated by a white triangle.

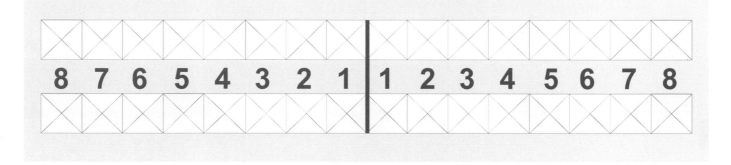

The Plaque Index can be calculated once these scores have been completed:

$$\frac{57 \text{ (number of areas with plaque)}}{128 \text{ (number of areas examined)}} \times 100 = 44.5\%$$

The Hygiene Index may be calculated in the same way, taking into consideration only the number of sites where there is no accumulation of plaque. This index accurately expresses patients' technical ability to clean their teeth.

In the presence of bleeding, a high Plaque Index indicates that plaque has been accumulating long enough to provoke inflammation. In the absence of bleeding, a high Plaque Index indicates that the accumulation is quite recent and that the patient has removed the plaque frequently enough to prevent inflammation.

Periodic verification of these indices is a valid way to identify areas that are still inflamed, making it possible to assess the patient's level of cooperation and the reaction of the tissues to periodontal therapy. It is not the percentage calculation that is important, but rather the assessment of both inflammation and the presence of plaque in the individual sites.

The methods described above, concomitant with examination of radiographic status, provide an accurate analysis of the presence, extent, and severity of periodontal disease. A correct diagnosis for each tooth supplies the basis for the treatment planning of each individual case.

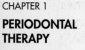

◤ OBJECTIVES OF PERIODONTAL THERAPY

The principal objective of periodontal therapy is to establish conditions that favor excellent plaque control to prevent the subgingival growth of bacterial deposits.[19]

This therapy develops in three phases:

> 1. **Cause-related therapy**
> 2. **Corrective therapy**
> 3. **Maintenance therapy**

1. The treatment of patients susceptible to periodontal disease begins with cause-related therapy, an initial phase of treatment aimed at the elimination of bacterial plaque, which is the cause of the disease.

2. Corrective therapy includes periodontal surgery, restorative treatment, endodontic treatment, and prosthodontic treatment. The goal of this therapy is to restore function and esthetics.

3. Lastly, maintenance therapy is the phase during which the patient, after the active therapy, undergoes periodic recalls. The goal of this phase is preventing, detecting, and treating recurrence of the disease as well as remotivating and reinstructing the patient whenever necessary.

▷ OBJECTIVES OF CAUSE-RELATED THERAPY

The goal of cause-related therapy is to eliminate supragingival and subgingival bacterial deposits and to prevent them from reaccumulating on the dental surfaces.

This treatment is one of the hygienist's principle tasks, and numerous studies have indicated that it should be accomplished by:

- **Motivation:** Encouraging the patient to combat periodontal disease

- **Self-performed oral hygiene** (Supragingival Plaque Control): Giving the patient instruction in the correct techniques of oral hygiene

- **Scaling and root planing** (Supragingival and Subgingival Instrumentation): Eliminating inflammation and stopping the progression of periodontal disease

Before dealing with these three aspects of cause-related therapy, a few considerations based on scientific findings should be made.

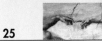
MOTIVATION: EFFECTS OF INFORMATION

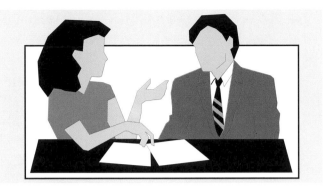

Many experts have studied the importance of information in motivating a patient.[2,12,13] The conclusion reached is that it is very important to give patients detailed information about their disease so that they become aware of their problem; this will lead patients to collaborate actively in the hygiene program that has been planned.

The subsequent oral hygiene appointments will be effective only if patients are aware of the importance that must be given to oral health.

Many long-term studies have compared the results obtained with different modalities of therapy (self-performed oral hygiene and/or scaling and root planing) performed alone or in concert.

EFFECTS OF SUPRAGINGIVAL PLAQUE CONTROL WITHOUT SUBGINGIVAL INSTRUMENTATION

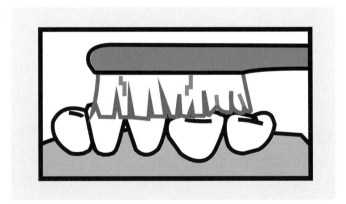

Contrasting results have been published regarding the effects obtained on the subgingival bacterial flora when control of supragingival plaque is performed without subgingival instrumentation. Where periodontitis was induced for experimental purposes in an animal model, findings proved that professional cleaning of the teeth repeated three times a week altered the quantity and the composition of the subgingival flora.[34]

Several studies carried out on human beings have confirmed the same results,[11,17,26,28,35] while others did not evidence the same effect.[8,14,18,22]

Differences in levels of plaque control and in the depth of pockets may account for these variable results. In fact, Dahlén et al[11] seem to indicate that carefully controlled oral hygiene in sites with pockets < 6 mm can greatly modify the quantity and composition of the subgingival flora. On the contrary, these effects were not observed in studies that included patients either with pockets that were > 6 mm[8] or where infrabony pockets were present.[16]

Therefore, in patients who present an advanced stage of periodontal disease, the control of supragingival plaque alone is not enough to prevent the progression of the disease.

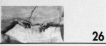

EFFECTS OF SUBGINGIVAL INSTRUMENTATION WITHOUT SUPRAGINGIVAL PLAQUE CONTROL

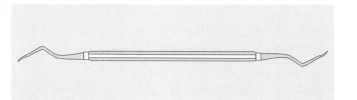

Some studies have assessed the effects of subgingival calculus removal and root planing that were not concomitant with appropriate self-performed plaque control on the part of patients themselves.[25,33]

From a microbiologic point of view, these studies have demonstrated that the bacterial flora present before treatment recolonized shortly after treatment. Therefore, these findings indicate that results obtained after subgingival instrumentation have a limited duration if they are not concomitant with an adequate control of supragingival plaque.

EFFECTS OF SUBGINGIVAL INSTRUMENTATION CONCOMITANT WITH SUPRAGINGIVAL PLAQUE CONTROL

From LIFE ART, 1998.
Reproduced with permission
of Lippincott/Williams & Wilkins

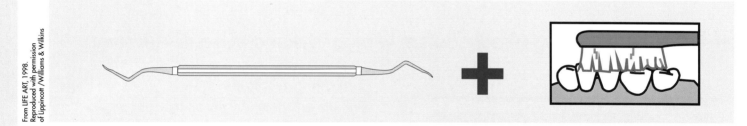

The efficacy of subgingival instrumentation concomitant with adequate supragingival plaque control in eliminating inflammation and arresting the progression of periodontal disease has been studied in numerous clinical trials.[3–7,10,15,23,24,27,29,31,36]

A series of clinical trials on single-rooted teeth assessed the efficacy of nonsurgical therapy on periodontal pockets varying in depth (from 5 to 12 mm).[4–7] After supragingival and subgingival instrumentation, a gradual but marked improvement in periodontal conditions was noted.

Furthermore, Badersten et al[7] studied the different results obtained by operators having varying levels of clinical experience in instrumentation (ranging from 3 to 14 years). The healing obtained by operators with varying levels of clinical experience was more or less the same.

In contrast, a study conducted by Brayer et al[9] compared the effects of subgingival instrumentation performed by more expert operators (periodontists) and those with less experience (general practioners specializing in periodontology). The results of this study showed that, especially in deep pockets, the expert operators removed a greater quantity of calculus than those who had not yet acquired the correct technique (less experienced operators). Therefore, in order to achieve maximum efficacy, it is important for the operator to acquire the correct technique of subgingival instrumentation.

EFFECTS OF SUBGINGIVAL INSTRUMENTATION IN DIFFERENT SITES

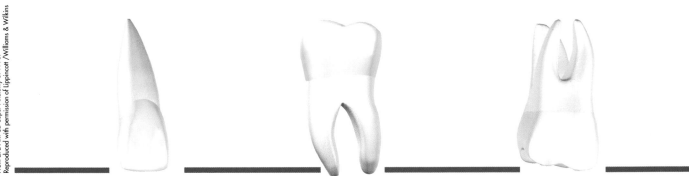

From LIFE ART 3D Super Anatomy 3. 1998. Reproduced with permission of Lippincott / Williams & Wilkins

Nordland et al[29] compared the effects of nonsurgical instrumentation on single-rooted teeth, on the smooth surfaces of molars, and in furcations. The findings showed that single-rooted teeth and smooth surfaces of molars healed comparably, while in furcations a higher percentage of sites lost further attachment. Other studies evidenced similar results.[22,32]

Therefore, with respect to other sites, furcations are more difficult to treat by nonsurgical instrumentation.

▶ SUMMARY

Self-performed oral hygiene measures alone are effective in resolving marginal gingivitis but have a limited or even no effect on subgingival plaque and signs of inflammation in deep periodontal pockets (> 6 mm). Therefore, in the treatment of periodontitis where deep pockets are present, plaque control alone will not produce noticeable results.

However, self-performed oral hygiene procedures concomitant with subgingival instrumentation are effective in:

1. Eliminating inflammation, even in deep pockets (especially around single-rooted teeth)
2. Reducing the probing depth in pockets
3. Improving the clinical attachment level

Finally, although the accessibility of the root surfaces is an essential factor in determining the results obtained by subgingival root instrumentation, the skill of the operator also has an important role in determining the success of the treatment.

▶ **REFERENCES**

1. Ainamo J, Bay I. Problems and proposals for recording gingivitis and plaque. Int Dent J 1975;25:229–235.

2. Alcouffe F. Improvement of oral hygiene habits: A psychological approach. J Clin Periodontol 1988;15:617–620.

3. Axelsson P, Lindhe J. Effect of controlled oral hygiene procedures on caries and periodontal disease in adults. J Clin Periodontol 1978;5:133–151.

4. Badersten A, Nilvéus R, Egelberg J. Effect of nonsurgical periodontal therapy. I. Moderately advanced periodontitis. J Clin Periodontol 1981;8:57–72.

5. Badersten A, Nilvéus R, Egelberg J. Effect of nonsurgical periodontal therapy. II. Severely advanced periodontitis. J Clin Periodontol 1984;11:63–76.

6. Badersten A, Nilvéus R, Egelberg J. Effect of nonsurgical periodontal therapy. III. Single versus repeated instrumentation. J Clin Periodontol 1984;11:114–124.

7. Badersten A, Nilvéus R, Egelberg J. Effect of non-surgical periodontal therapy (IV). Operator variability. J Clin Periodontol 1985;12:190–200.

8. Beltrami M, Bickel M, Baehni PC. The effect of supragingival plaque control on the composition of the subgingival microflora in human periodontitis. J Clin Periodontol 1987;14:161–164.

9. Brayer WK, Mellonig JT, Dunlap RM, Marinak KW, Carson RE. Scaling and root planing effectiveness: The effect of root surface access and operator experience. J Periodontol 1989;60:67–72.

10. Cercek JF, Kiger RD, Garrett S, Egelberg J. Relative effects of plaque control and instrumentation on the clinical parameters of human periodontal disease. J Clin Periodontol 1983;10:46–56.

11. Dahlén G, Lindhe J, Sato K, Hanamura H, Okamoto H. The effect of supragingival plaque control on the subgingival microbiota in subjects with periodontal disease. J Clin Periodontol 1992;19: 802–809.

12. Emler BF, Windchy AM, Zaino SW, Feldman SM, Scheetz JP. The value of repetition and reinforcement in improving oral hygiene performance. J Periodontol 1980;51:228–234.

13. Glavind L. Means and methods in oral hygiene instruction of adults. A review. Tandlægebladet 1990;94:211–246.

14. Greenwell H, Bakr A, Bissada N, Debanne S, Rowland D. The effect of Keyes' method of oral hygiene on the subgingival microflora compared to the effect of scaling and/or surgery. J Clin Periodontol 1985;12:327–341.

15. Hämmerle CHF, Joss A, Lang NP. Short-term effects of initial periodontal therapy (hygienic phase). J Clin Periodontol 1991;18:233–239.

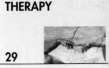

16. Hellström MK, Ramberg P, Krok L, Lindhe J. The effect of supragingival plaque control on the subgingival microflora in human periodontitis. J Clin Periodontol 1996;23:934–940.

17. Katsanoulas T, Reneè I, Attström R. The effect of supragingival plaque control on the composition of the subgingival flora in periodontal pockets. J Clin Periodontol 1992;19:760–765.

18. Kho P, Smales FC, Hardie JM. The effect of supragingival plaque control on the subgingival microflora. J Clin Periodontol 1985;12:676–686.

19. Lindhe J. Clinical Periodontology and Implant Dentistry, ed 3. Copenhagen: Munksgaard, 1997:chap 12, 15, 26.

20. Lindhe J, Hamp SE, Löe H. Plaque induced periodontal disease in beagle dogs. A 4-year clinical, roentgenographical and histometrical study. J Periodontal Res 1975;10:243–255.

21. Löe H, Theilade E, Jensen SB. Experimental gingivitis in man. J Periodontol 1965;36:177–187.

22. Loos B, Claffey N, Crigger M. Effects of oral hygiene measures on clinical and microbiological parameters of periodontal disease. J Clin Periodontol 1988;15:211–216.

23. Loos B, Nylund K, Claffey N, Egelberg J. Clinical effects of root debridement in molar and non-molar teeth: A 2-year follow-up. J Clin Periodontol 1989;16:498–504.

24. Lovdal A, Arno A, Schei O, Waerhaug J. Combined effect of subgingival scaling and root planing and controlled oral hygiene on the incidence of gingivitis. Acta Odontol Scand 1961;19: 537–555.

25. Magnusson I, Lindhe J, Yoneyama T, Liljenberg B. Recolonization of a subgingival microbiota following scaling in deep pockets. J Clin Periodontol 1984;11:193–207.

26. McNabb H, Mombelli A, Lang NP. Supragingival cleaning 3 times a week. J Clin Periodontol 1992;19:348–356.

27. Morrison EC, Ramfjörd SP, Hill RW. Short-term effects of initial, nonsurgical periodontal treatment (hygienic phase). J Clin Periodontol 1980;7:199–211.

28. Müller HP, Hartmann J, Flores-de-Jacoby L. Clinical alterations in relation to the morphological composition of the subgingival microflora following scaling and root planing. J Clin Periodontol 1986;13:825–832.

29. Nordland P, Garrett S, Kiger R, Vanooteghem R, Hutchens LH, Egelberg J. The effect of plaque control and root debridement in molar teeth. J Clin Periodontol 1987;14:231–236.

30. O'Leary TJ, Drake RB, Naylor JE. The plaque control record. J Periodontol 1972;43:38.

31. Proye M, Caton J, Polson A. Initial healing of periodontal pockets after a single episode of root planing monitored by controlled probing forces. J Periodontol 1982;53:296–301.

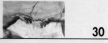
32. Ramfjörd SP, Caffesse RG, Morrison EC, et al. Four modalities of periodontal treatment compared over 5 years. J Clin Periodontol 1987;14:445–452.

33. Sbordone L, Ramaglia L, Gulletta E, Iacono V. Recolonization of the subgingival microflora after scaling and root planing in human periodontitis. J Periodontol 1990;61:579–584.

34. Siegrist B, Kornman KS. The effect of supragingival plaque control on the composition of the subgingival microbial flora in ligature-induced periodontitis in the monkey. J Dent Res 1982;61: 936–941.

35. Smulow JB, Turesky SS, Hill RG. The effect of supragingival plaque removal on anaerobic bacteria in deep periodontal pockets. J Am Dent Assoc 1983;107:737–742.

36. Suomi JD, Green JC, Vermillion JR, Doyle J, Chang JJ, Leatherwood EC. The effect of controlled oral hygiene procedures on the progression of periodontal disease in adults. Results after third and final year. J Periodontol 1971;42:152–160.

EXPERIENCE
IS THE BEST TEACHER

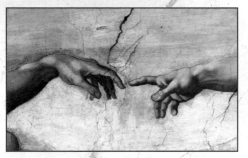

CHAPTER 2

MOTIVATION

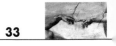
WHAT DOES "MOTIVATING" A PATIENT MEAN?

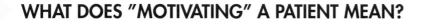

When periodontally compromised patients arrive at the surgery, they are first examined by the dentist, who establishes the treatment plan and advises them to make a series of appointments with the hygienist for the required sittings of oral hygiene. Often, when patients meet the hygienist, they do not clearly understand the type of treatment they must undergo, how it will be performed and, above all, the role they themselves will have in determining the success of the treatment.

The term "motivation" means conveying to the patient, through a series of words, gestures, and examples, the importance that self-performed oral hygiene has in the health of the oral cavity.

In order to achieve this goal, hygienists must possess:

- **Technical skill**
- **Communication skill**
- **Psychologic insight**

During my years in the profession, I have met and treated many patients. This has given me the opportunity not only to observe many different clinical aspects of their pathologies, but also to become acquainted with a wide range of personalities and mentalities. I have come to realize that there is no single approach that can be used successfully to motivate all patients. In fact, after carefully evaluating their disease, many factors involving their personal backgrounds must also be taken into consideration. I am convinced that you must really understand your patients in order to motivate them.

Occasionally, at the end of my courses, I have been surprised to receive favorable comments regarding advice given to help operators perform various aspects of their work more easily. Initially, I was hesitant to voice these suggestions because I considered them very simple, personal, and not necessarily interesting or helpful for everyone; but, to my great pleasure, experience proved the contrary and eventually encouraged me to offer these suggestions to others in this text. My intention is not to establish a series of rules or a fixed pattern to follow, indicating them as "the best." I would simply like to offer advice and opinions based on my personal experience.

Hygienists may have great technical skill, perform scaling and root planing properly, and be perfectly acquainted with the instruments necessary for self-performed oral hygiene, but they will not succeed in their profession if they are unable to communicate with their patients in order to motivate them. Therefore, psychologic insight is both helpful and necessary in order to perceive patients' problems, needs, anxieties, fears, bad habits, and lifestyles.

Using the method that they consider the most appropriate for the case in question, hygienists should offer suggestions that are both easy to follow and helpful in guiding patients to choose the most convenient moment for their self-performed oral hygiene so that it does not become a torment or a burden. They should also be sympathetic to patients' reality and problems, stimulating in order to involve them, and spontaneous and enthusiastic to facilitate the establishment of a good relationship. Self-control and calm are also essential during possible discussions or misunderstandings.

Lastly, hygienists must take great care of their personal appearance, which should be plain but pleasant, with a fresh uniform. I advise women to avoid showy rings or jewelry, to use light makeup, and to adopt a neat hairstyle. I advise men to present themselves cleanly shaven or with their beards well trimmed. And, of course, both male and female hygienists must always have clean teeth!

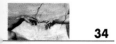

FUNDAMENTAL BEHAVIOR

In order to motivate the patient, the hygienist must exhibit:

> **1. Willingness**
> **2. Professional Self-Confidence**

WILLINGNESS

There must be adequate time at the hygienist's disposal in order to motivate the patient. The telephone or other interruptions must not interfere with the hygienist's concentration on the patient being treated.

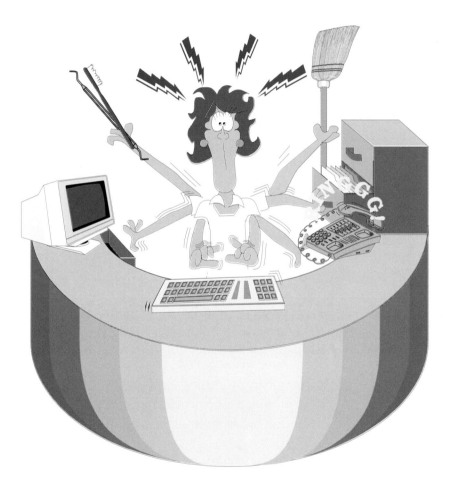

Patients will not pay attention to any information unless they are aware that the hygienist is really interested in the case. The hygienist should consider the patient's fears and problems and should try to establish an individual relationship with each person treated. This relationship will eventually lead to mutual understanding, and may even develop into friendship.

PROFESSIONAL SELF-CONFIDENCE

During the first dental examination, periodontally compromised patients are informed that periodontal treatment that generally begins with several hygiene appointments will be required; therefore, when patients arrive they may already have basic ideas about oral hygiene. Some patients may even have doubts about the real necessity of having to undergo "so many appointments" that might cost them more than necessary! The hygienist's task is to make the patient understand why this particular treatment is necessary; therefore, the hygienist's image must convey self-confidence and a sincere interest in the patient's problem.

The hygienist must try to have an answer for everything, proving to be prepared and competent. At times, the hygienist may also have to tolerate patients' irritating comments and make them understand that the treatment is necessary in order to solve their problems in the best possible way.

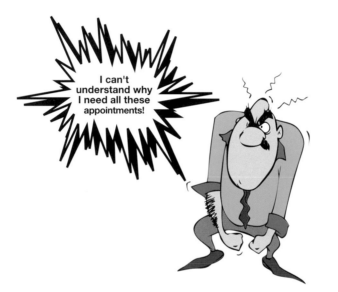

The hygienist should realize that a patient may never have been to the dentist before or may never have undergone such a particular and meticulous treatment.

Patients must love their teeth; this is the fact that will make them willing to listen and collaborate.

COMMUNICATING WITH THE PATIENT

In the attempt to establish a relationship based on mutual trust, which is fundamental for the success of treatment, the hygienist must strive to reduce the patient's apprehension and discover the causes of it through a friendly and open dialogue. The hygienist should become a friendly figure, a trusted person who serves as a link between the patient and the medical staff, establishing a relationship that may help to allay the patient's fear and apprehension about the dentist. The latter may not always have the time to apply an adequate psychologic approach and will benefit from finding a patient who is relaxed, prepared, and collaborative.[5]

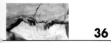

Experience has taught me to apply some simple psychologic strategies, which I present here as suggestions that may be used to facilitate dialogue with the patient during motivation.

• Begin communication by greeting patients cordially and calling them by name to "personalize" the relationship that is to be established.

• Communicate with patients using simple, comprehensible words that enable explanations and instructions to be understood easily. In this regard, an outline may be prepared in advance so that the hygienist will not have to improvise and risk neglecting important subjects.

• Attempt to direct the conversation toward subjects that stimulate patients' interest.

• Show interest in what patients say and induce them to analyze and comment on their own behavior. This strategy can, in fact, lead to important results: On the one hand, patients are encouraged to "confide" in the person who is paying so much attention; on the other hand, the hygienist is able to discover how much patients already know about their problem and to perceive, at the same time, any eventual inadequacies in the message conveyed.

• Create a reassuring atmosphere that can help to reduce patients' anxiety, demonstrating that what they say and feel is entirely understandable.

• Lead patients to change their attitude. Never openly contradict patients, but guide them to discover their own mistakes. Encouragement always gets better results than criticism. Thus, at the end of the conversation, patients will decide if they want to do something for their teeth without feeling coerced into doing so, but will be aware that they have made the right decision.

• To avoid a regression of the hygienist-patient relationship, never accuse, frighten, or offend patients.

• Take advantage of, and utilize, patients' positive feelings, pointing out their own abilities. Patients must acquire self-confidence and understand that they can do a lot for their own dental health.

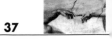

• Be careful not to overburden patients by giving too much information all at once, and always make sure that the explanations given have been clearly understood to avoid "estrangement." The length of the conversation must be established according to each patient's level of education, social level, and emotional state.

• Use a system of personal diagnosis, showing patients their own plaque level colored by the plaque-disclosing agents, the bleeding of their own gingiva, the insertion of the probe in their own periodontal pockets, and their own radiographic situation.

• Substantiate the explanation with scientific proof that is inherent to the case being treated, but presented according to the patient's level of education.

• Prearrange and maintain a suitable environment, selecting with care comfortable chairs, adequate lighting, furniture with pleasant colors, and a well-adjusted room temperature.

In brief, do not conduct the conversation with the patient as if it were an interrogation or a series of illogical questions. The efforts to perceive patients' expectations, fears, and emotions are intended to stimulate the patients' awareness, which is indispensable for a constructive motivation.

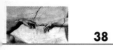

SUBJECTS OF DISCUSSION DURING MOTIVATION

CONSULTATION OF THE STOMATOLOGIC CLINICAL CHART

• Case history
• First examination

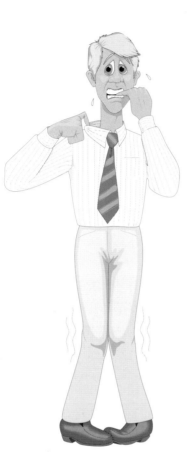

Initially, it is better to have the patient sit on a comfortable chair in front of a mirror rather than on the dentist's chair; this helps to put the patient at ease, thus facilitating the hygienist's attempt to communicate and establish a good relationship. This approach is opportune, above all, for those patients who are particularly anxious and afraid of the dentist's chair; patients will be reassured by the fact that as long as they are seated in the armchair, no "drill" will be used. Substantially, our motivation is a chat that gradually leads the patient to relax.

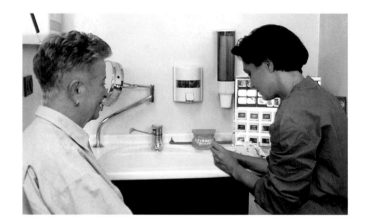

Together with the patient, the hygienist examines the clinical chart, which contains important information such as the patient's occupation, the referring person, case history, and any previous periodontal treatment. It is important to know patients' occupations in order to have an idea of their cultural level and lifestyle.

It is also important to know who may have referred patients, because if they have been sent by another person who is already under treatment at the dental office—and is therefore already motivated—we will benefit from this, given that even if we do not know the patient yet, the patient knows us indirectly.

The analysis of the patients' case histories makes it possible to evaluate their state of health and to act accordingly. Moreover, it is very important to know if the patient has undergone previous periodontal therapy. If this is the case, and the patient still has problems, it is evident that the prior treatment was not successful and it is therefore necessary to discover the reasons for its failure.

The motivation will be based on the various problems that emerge; any diseases indicated should be discussed, encouraging patients to offer information spontaneously. The treatment plan prepared by the dentist after the first examination will allow organization of the required oral hygiene appointments.

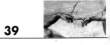

We should pay particular attention to the periodontal clinical charts that have already been compiled and to the radiographic and photographic status of patients so that we will be immediately aware of their situation.

INITIAL EXAMINATION — R. G. 63

Tooth	m	b	d	l	Furc Inv	Mob
18	?	?	?	?		
17	5*		5*	4*		
16	5*	5*	5*		B1	
15	5*		5*			
14	5*		5*			
13	6*		5*			
12	6*		6*			1
11	5*		8*	8*		2
21	5*		6*			
22	6*		5*			
23	5*		4*			
24	5*		5*			
25						
26	5*	5*	5*	5*		
27	5*		8*			1
28	11*	9*	6*	5*		2

Tooth	m	b	d	l	Furc Inv	Mob
48	6*		5*	4*		
47	5*		8*			
46						
45	9*		4*			
44	5		8*	7*		2
43	8*		6*			
42	6*		6*			
41	6*	5*	8*			2
31	8*	5*	7*	4*		2
32	6*		6*			
33	5*		5*			
34	6*		4*	4*		
35	4*		4*			
36	4*		4*			
37						
38						

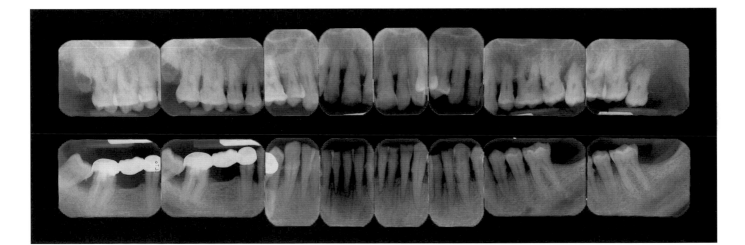

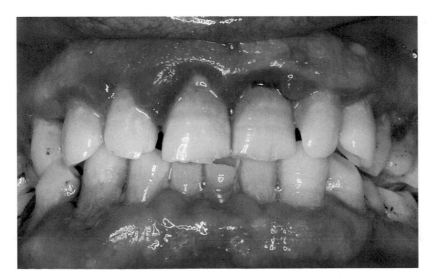

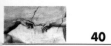

INFORMATION ABOUT CARIES AND PERIODONTAL DISEASE: HOW TO EXPLAIN THE DISEASE TO THE PATIENT

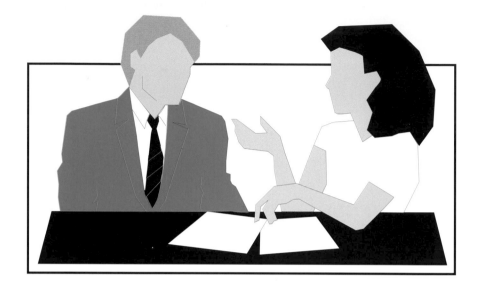

It is now necessary to explain the causes of caries and periodontal disease to the patient; understanding the disease is the most important thing.[6] In order to supply comprehensible information, the hygienist must have a thorough knowledge of these two pathologies so that they can be explained as simply as possible, avoiding the use of technical terminology. If the patient is a doctor, or has basic scientific knowledge, the explanation may be given in scientific terms.

It is very difficult to find the right words to explain the problem adequately to the patient. There is a risk of being too scientific, either using words that are too complex for the patient or going into the explanation too deeply so that the patient becomes bored. On the other hand, we may oversimplify, making it difficult for the patient to understand the course of disease. Thus, we must try to give all the essential information in simple terms so that the patient is aware of and understands the problem.

The subject of periodontal disease is particularly complex because patients often have no knowledge of it. Many times I have heard patients say: "I'm fine. I don't have even one cavity and I've never had a toothache!" while perhaps they are losing their teeth because of periodontitis and are not aware of it.

During my years of professional experience, I have met very few patients who have proven to have sufficient knowledge of this disease or of the correct technique for brushing. Those who had previously undergone periodontal treatment knew about the problem, but the majority were convinced that sooner or later the disease would recur. Very few of them knew that they should have followed a maintenance program after active therapy.

HOW TO MOTIVATE A PERIODONTAL PATIENT

A plastic model and a periodontal probe can be used to illustrate various aspects of the disease; atlases and booklets may also be useful for the same purpose.

I devised a booklet in which I illustrate and explain, in simple terms, all of the fundamental aspects of periodontal disease. In addition to the plastic model, I use the photos and drawings of this booklet to facilitate my explanation of the progression of the disease. I give the booklet to the patient when the appointment is over so that the concepts that I explained can be read about at home in order to better assimilate and understand them.

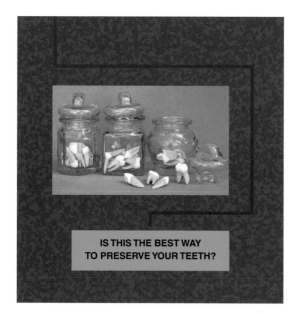

IS THIS THE BEST WAY
TO PRESERVE YOUR TEETH?

After explaining the disease, it is important to disclose the patients' plaque and show them their own periodontal pockets and radiographs in order to gain their interest.

The information that patients must receive about the causes and symptoms of periodontal disease may be given in various ways. The "gradual system," which has been used for many years in a great number of cases treated at the Department of Periodontology of the University of Göteborg in Sweden,[2-4] follows this outline:

Explain to patients in simple words:
1. The cause of periodontal disease
2. What can be done to cure it
3. What can be done to prevent it from recurring

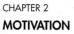
SIMULATION OF A DIRECT DIALOGUE WITH A PATIENT

In the following section, the text in italics exemplifies the simple, illustrative language that I use when communicating with patients. The images included in this simulation are provided to help the reader remember what must be explained to patients.

THE CAUSE OF PERIODONTAL DISEASE

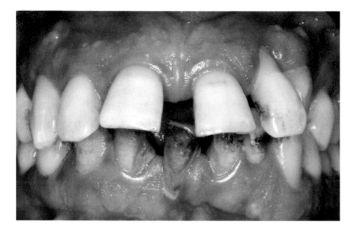

"Periodontitis is a disease that affects the gums and all the areas surrounding the tooth, unlike caries, which affects the tooth itself.

"Both caries and inflammation of the gums are caused by bacterial plaque. Bacterial plaque is an extremely complex deposit of sticky bacteria that clings firmly to the tooth.

"It is normal to have bacteria in the mouth, but if they are not removed every day with a toothbrush, those that have deposited stubbornly on the tooth can cause caries.

"The sugar in our diet nourishes the bacteria, causing them to release acids that corrode the enamel of the tooth.

"Bacteria that have penetrated into the sulcus between the tooth and the gum may inflame the gum itself. This condition, if neglected, may cause tooth loss."

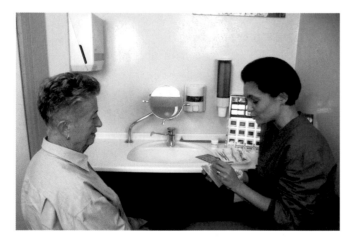

As I am speaking, I indicate the gingival sulcus using a periodontal probe on a plastic model.

Patients susceptible to caries will receive particular instructions regarding correct dietary habits, fluoride prophylaxis, home care, and periodic recalls. I have noticed that patients are better acquainted with caries than with periodontal disease; therefore, with periodontally compromised patients it is necessary to give more detailed information.

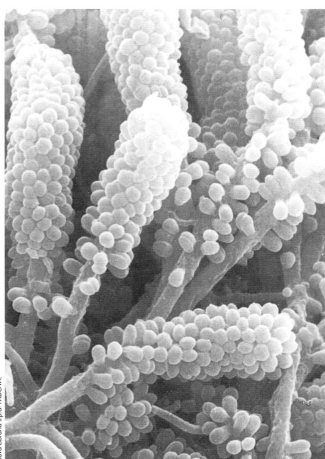

From "Atlante di Odontoiatria" directed by K.H. Rateischak - N. 4 Carioprofilassi e Terapia Conservativa - Peter Reithe in collaboration with Gunther Rau - Piccin Nuova Libraria s.p.a. PADOVA.

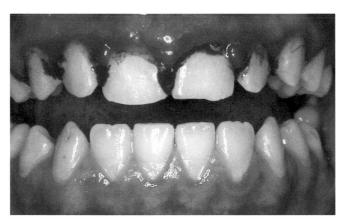

"Normally, in a healthy mouth, the sulcus is approximately 1 to 1.5 mm deep. The bacteria penetrate into this gap and cling firmly to the tooth and to one another, organizing themselves like a cob of corn. Then, they begin to release toxic substances that are similar to poisons.

"The body reacts to the presence of these bacteria by sending blood cells that are able to combat these microbes. That is why gums bleed! Healthy gums must not bleed!"

At this point, patients might say that they thought gingival bleeding was a positive factor. In fact, there is a widespread belief that bleeding is a sign of healthy gingiva. I clarify that this is a misinterpretation and I continue the motivation, explaining that:

"Bleeding is one of the body's natural defenses, and it is a good thing that it intervenes. Otherwise, the bacteria could cause tooth loss. However, it is also a warning sign that clearly indicates where the plaque has accumulated."

Patients should recognize bleeding as the first indication of a problem. From this moment on, they will know what to do when the problem occurs.

"If you see your gums bleeding, you should not stop brushing your teeth. It is not your toothbrush that is provoking the bleeding. You must continue brushing, using the correct technique to disrupt and remove the plaque that is causing the bleeding.

"Naturally, for a certain period, the body's defenses are able to combat the attack of microbes that tend to penetrate in depth. This is referred to as marginal inflammation of the gums, which in technical terms is called 'gingivitis.'

"Patients may have gingivitis all of their lives and the condition may never worsen because the natural defenses are able to keep the plaque under control. But sometimes other problems set in.

"As time passes, if the plaque is not disrupted, it may become laden with more dangerous microorganisms that can release toxic substances. These substances may in turn destroy the fibers that keep the gum attached to the bone and the tooth. At the same time, periods of weakness in our body's natural defenses may facilitate the growth of bacteria."

As I continue the explanation, I try to illustrate certain concepts using the periodontal probe on the plastic model.

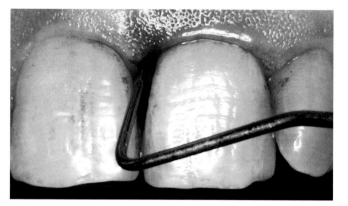

"Due to this accumulation of bacteria, the sulcus becomes a pocket that may deepen to 4, 6, 8, or even 10 mm.

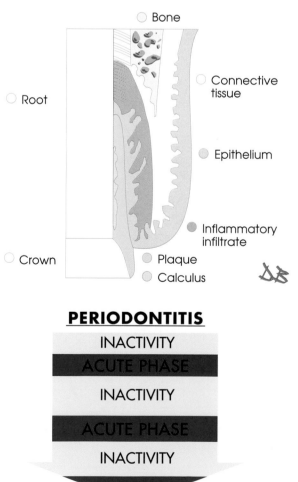

Bone

Connective tissue

Root

Epithelium

Inflammatory infiltrate

Crown

Plaque

Calculus

"This is called periodontal disease.

PERIODONTITIS

INACTIVITY

ACUTE PHASE

INACTIVITY

ACUTE PHASE

INACTIVITY

LOSS OF ATTACHMENT

"The course of periodontal disease is usually very slow, characterized by periods of inactivity and periods of acute inflammation.

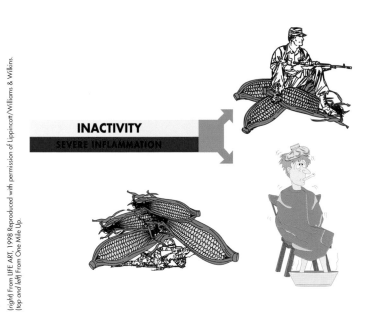

INACTIVITY

SEVERE INFLAMMATION

"In periods of inactivity, which may be quite long, the body's natural defenses are able to block the advancement of the bacteria. The gums bleed less and are less inflamed and the situation does not worsen.

"During periods of severe inflammation, which are usually shorter, the body's defenses cannot control all the bacteria that are present. This is either because the quantity of the bacteria has increased, causing the pocket to deepen, or because the defenses are weakened as a result of, for example, the presence of another disease. During this period, the gums may appear very red and swollen and may bleed a lot, at times even spontaneously."

After this explanation, patients generally confirm that they had in fact also noticed this cycle but in the moments of inactivity thought that the gingiva had healed. In the meantime, years have passed!

At this point, it is time to approach the subject of tooth mobility, trying to make it simple for patients to understand.

"As the battle between bacteria and natural defenses continues, the deepening of the pockets is accompanied by the destruction of the bone of the upper and lower jaws. Because it is the bone, not the gums, that holds teeth in place, the destruction of this bone can cause very serious damage.

"Try to imagine a skull. The teeth are inserted in holes in the bone, which gives them stability.

"When the gum surrounds the tooth, it protects the bone underneath. However, in cases in which the gum is pulled away from the tooth in certain areas, it no longer protects the bone, which is now vulnerable to damage by bacteria.

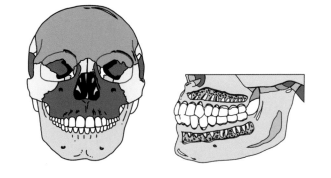

"Therefore, the stability of a tooth is determined by the amount of bone that supports that tooth.

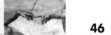
"As the bone is destroyed, the tooth first becomes loose and, in the course of time, falls out. This is the outcome of periodontal disease.

"A tooth is like a lamp post set in the ground: If you remove the earth around it, the lamp post falls down!

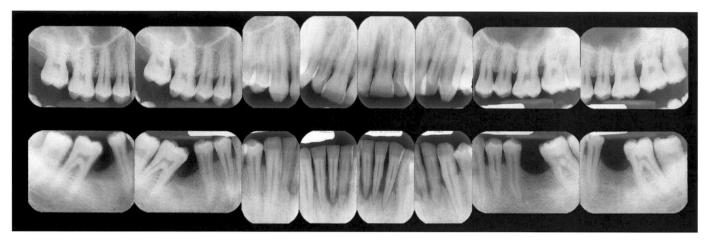

"Years ago, all patients affected by this disease could do nothing but wait for their teeth to fall out.

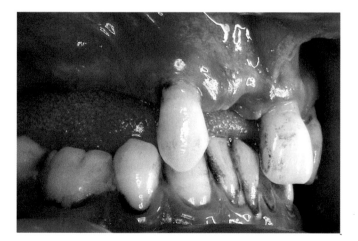
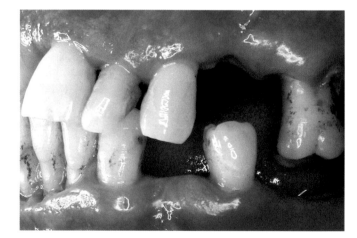

"Now, many things can be done, even if some bone has been destroyed.

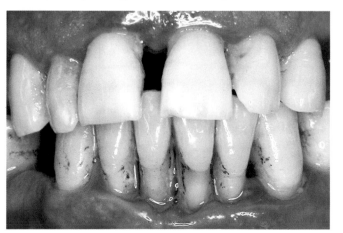
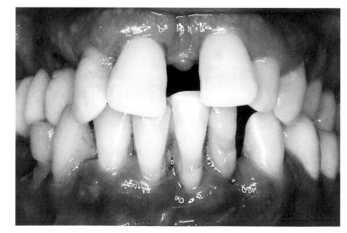

"Unfortunately, however, very little can be done once the bone has disappeared."

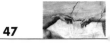

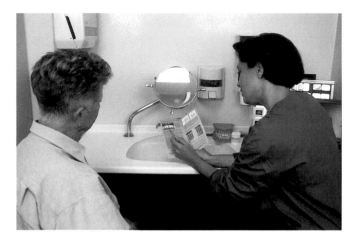

Up until this point, I have given the patient a general description of periodontal disease, the main aspects of which are summarized in my booklet. Together with the patient, I look at the illustrations and photos and emphasize the most important aspects.

I then begin to personalize the topic by introducing the clinical data related to the patient's own disease. The patient is curious to know how much bone has been lost and how much remains.

We look at the clinical chart on which the results of the probing of the patient's own periodontal pockets are recorded, and then we examine the patient's own radiographs.

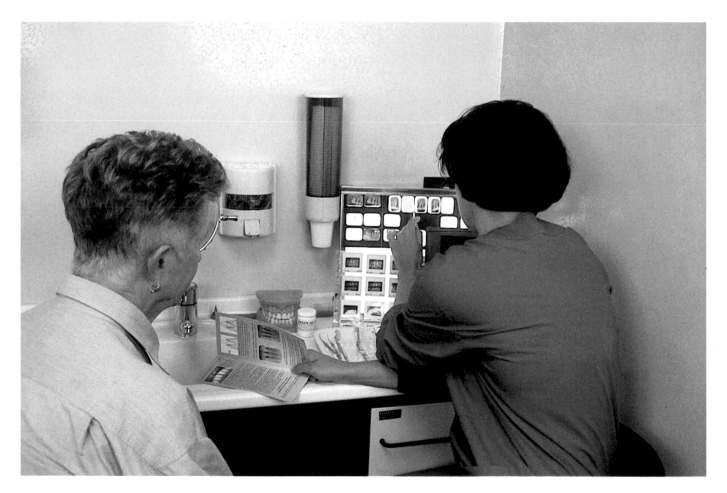

Patients usually appear to be very interested because they are receiving information that is for the most part new and that, above all, concerns their personal condition.

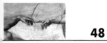

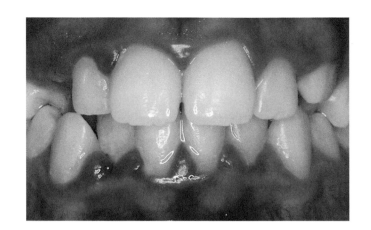

"At this point, you can understand that everything started from simple gingivitis, a marginal inflammation of the gums caused by plaque. If we remove these bacteria immediately, the gums become healthy again. Gingivitis heals in a few days!

"Therefore, periodontal disease can be prevented. It is not a hereditary disease, but you can inherit the tendency to be susceptible to the particular plaque that can attack the gums.

"No doubt you know people who have never brushed their teeth and yet, even at a certain age, have all their teeth! They are lucky because they have good natural defenses and the conditions in their mouth are not suitable for the plaque to become dangerous. You must not compare yourself to these people because your mouth does provide a good environment for bacteria that can trigger the disease."

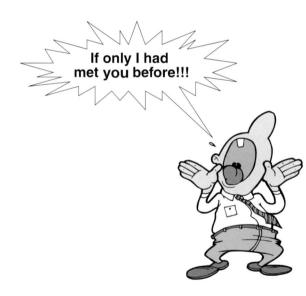

If only I had met you before!!!

I evaluate my communication skills at this moment. If patients have understood my message correctly, they will probably tell me that if they had learned to perform correct oral hygiene previously, they would surely have been able to keep their own teeth in good condition.

I never forget that my task is to make patients aware of the problem so that they will draw their own conclusions without my prompting.

In many cases, I find that it is helpful to alert patients that periodontal disease may also affect younger members of the family.

"Seeing that there is a predisposition to this problem in your family, I advise you to check your children's teeth. Look carefully to see if their gums bleed. If you notice this symptom, they must learn to clean their teeth properly, and they should also be examined by a dentist."

I think it is necessary to make parents feel responsible for their children's teeth. I try to offer suggestions that can help them avoid periodontis, at least for the younger members of their family. Patients appreciate this consideration very much.

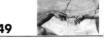

CURING PERIODONTAL DISEASE

"If there is only gingivitis, then the damage is superficial. In this case, the appropriate oral hygiene, which I am going to teach you, plus a few professional cleanings will solve the problem in a few weeks and the gums will stop bleeding and become healthy again.

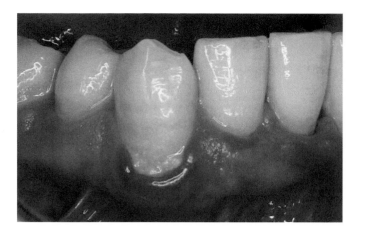
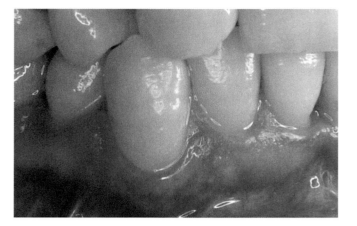

"The oral hygiene appointments are necessary to remove tartar. Tartar is hardened plaque that can no longer be removed with a toothbrush alone. During these appointments, your teeth will also be polished and specific products will be applied if your teeth are hypersensitive to hot or cold or the touch of a toothbrush.

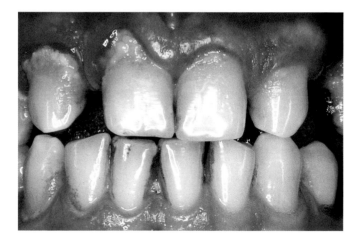
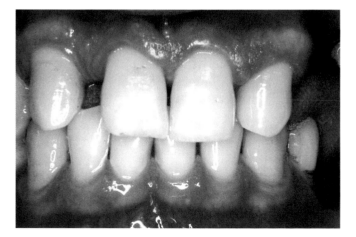

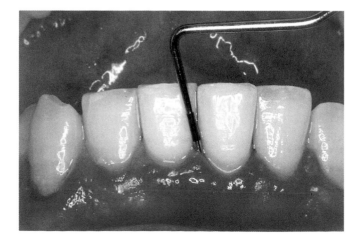

"If the damage is more than superficial and there are pockets, cleaning the sulcus is not enough. In this case, it is necessary to clean in depth, under the gum, with particular instruments that are designed to remove plaque and tartar.

"This will give the gums a chance to heal. Naturally, you will be given local anesthesia so that you will not feel any pain. This is the only way that I will be able to clean as deep as possible."

In giving this information to the patient, it is important to weigh the fact that expert hygienists will be able to treat and heal deeper pockets than will others who have less experience. Therefore, operators must be aware of their own technical skills when emphasizing the effectiveness of nonsurgical scaling.

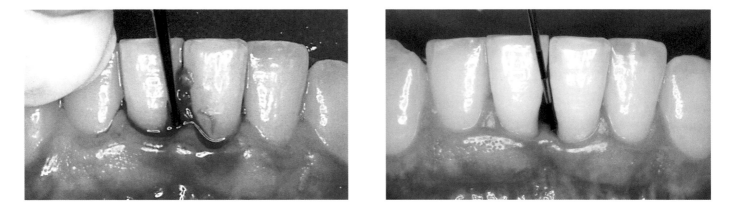

At this point, I continue the motivation, supplying simple explanations to help the patient understand the various treatments that may be necessary and emphasizing the importance of self-performed oral hygiene.

"Your collaboration at home is fundamental. I will teach you how to use the instruments that I recommend so that you can carry out correct oral hygiene, which is essential to the success of the treatment. If you do not do your part, there will not be a noticeable improvement when you return for a reevaluation after a few months.

"Otherwise, after a few months, thanks mostly to your efforts, the dentist will find your mouth in good condition. At this point, the majority of the pockets should be completely healed and if a few remain, they should be notably reduced in size.

"However, you should know that in some areas the teeth might appear a little longer after the gums have healed, especially where the disease has destroyed more bone. This may be a slight disadvantage from an esthetic point of view, but the important thing is to interrupt the course of the disease. If you follow my instructions, together we will achieve our goal."

The patient must understand that their commitment to collaborate is a fundamental contribution toward the success of the treatment.

"When you return to the dentist for your reevaluation, you may be told that the situation has improved and that the gums do not require surgical treatment. Or, on the contrary, you may hear that some pockets are still present and have not healed. Why?

"One reason may be that you have not been thorough enough at home, and as a result there may still be deposits of plaque and the gums may not yet be healed. In this case, you will return to me and we will try to improve the situation.

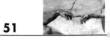

"Or, you may have cleaned your teeth very well, as I hope, but a small quantity of tartar may be left at the bottom of some pockets that therefore have not healed. In this case, the dentist may decide to have me make a further attempt at cleaning the pockets. Or, it may be necessary to perform surgery, opening the gum and cleaning the sites I was not able to reach. This operation is tolerable because it is not particularly painful and it does not cause problems afterward.

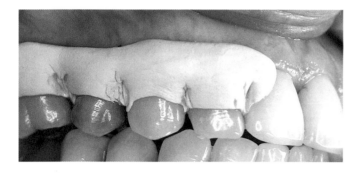

"Sometimes, in order to protect the wound, it may be necessary to apply a dressing, the 'plaster' that is used in the mouth...

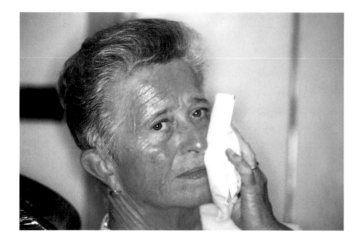

"...and an ice pack may be utilized to limit possible swelling.

"Furthermore, while you are healing, we will help to keep the wound clean."

If I note that the treatment plan organized by the dentist already indicates that periodontal surgery is necessary in some areas, I usually inform the patient that:

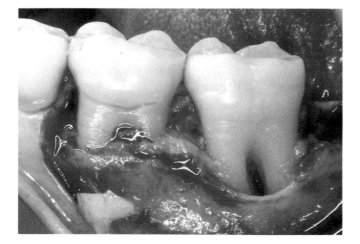

"The dentist has already decided that surgery is necessary in some areas of your mouth. This means that there is an initial situation that I cannot resolve. A few preliminary hygiene appointments are, however, necessary in order to clean these areas, at least marginally, and to prepare the tissue for surgery.

"I also have to teach you how to take care of your mouth and keep it clean. Unfortunately, if you don't do your part, the operation will be useless."

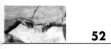

PREVENTING PERIODONTAL DISEASE FROM RECURRING

I approach prevention of recurrence of periondontal disease by telling the patient that:

"Our aim is not just to cure your disease, but also to prevent it from coming back. The success of the treatment depends on you and your willingness to do your part.

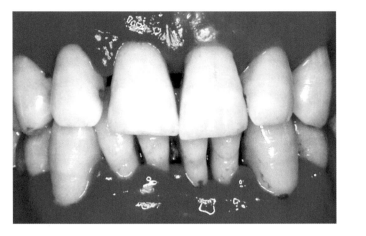
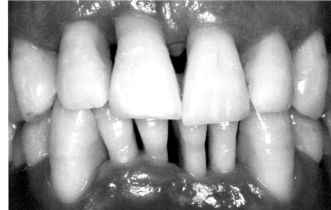

"When everything has been resolved, I advise you to return for periodic checkups to maintain the health of your mouth.

"If you don't disrupt the plaque every day, you will have a relapse. We have changed the health status of your mouth, but the harmful bacteria that make up your plaque still have the potential to cause serious damage. If you continue your home care diligently, I should find your oral cavity quite clean when you return for a checkup.

"If this is the case, I will not have to repeat the treatment and will only have to verify that everything is proceeding well. If necessary, I will show you the areas that are still inflamed so that you can clean them more carefully.

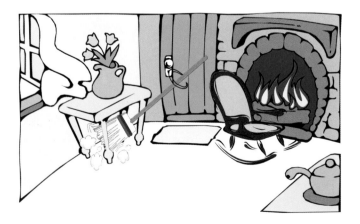

"Think of your mouth as a house. Initially, my task is to clean this house well for you and to teach you how to keep it tidy using the proper equipment. After a few months, if you have cleaned this house every day, what will remain to be done? Perhaps there will be a little dust in the corners, but on the whole it should be very clean. In much the same way, if you clean your mouth thoroughly every day, when you return for a checkup I should have little or no cleaning to do. At most, I may have to touch up the areas of your mouth that are difficult for you to reach."

Calling the patient's attention to specific areas means giving the patient the responsibility of keeping them checked and clean.

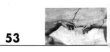

Once I have clarified the patient's responsibilities, I give further information about my professional role:

"If we proceed this way, you are very unlikely to have a recurrence of the disease. Once the work has been done, I will only have to organize periodic checkups. I will not have to perform further scaling. Tartar only forms if you allow the plaque time to harden.

"I am here to help you and can offer advice whenever you need it, but you must realize that the success of the treatment depends above all on your ability to maintain a good level of oral hygiene. Your teeth may be perfectly clean and therefore you may need me only rarely. However, if your mouth is not in perfect condition, I will have to help you to reach the sites that you haven't been able to clean adequately.

"As time passes, you may become less attentive in cleaning your mouth. When you come for a checkup, I will not only clean your teeth but I will have the opportunity to renew your enthusiasm and to remind you that your cooperation is very important. If you show that you have been very thorough and are able to carry on by yourself, I will tell you to come less often for checkups. The frequency of these checkups will therefore depend on how meticulous you are in performing your oral hygiene."

It is important to mention maintenance therapy from the first appointment because in this way patients, who are now aware of the problem, understand that the hygienist is there to help them, even after active therapy has concluded. Patients need protection. However, they must not put themselves entirely in the hands of the hygienist, because they have to remain active and collaborative.

At this point, the following instructions, related to the techniques of oral hygiene, will be effective because the patient is now aware that oral health is very important and that the goal must be to obtain it and maintain it.

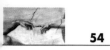

EDUCATING THE PATIENT IN SELF-PERFORMED ORAL HYGIENE

Once patients understand the problem, it is necessary to teach them how to clean the oral cavity.

The patient should be very "angry" with the plaque and ready to defeat it.

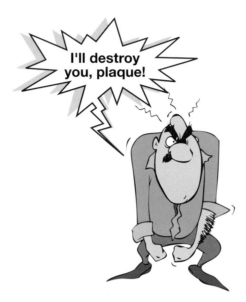

It may be useful to disclose patients' plaque by means of a disclosing agent in order to help them understand their hygiene situation.

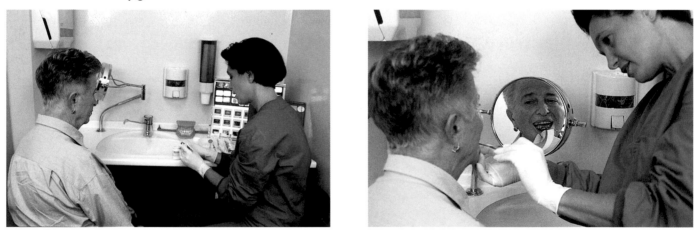

It is important that patients realize for themselves that their oral hygiene is not sufficient.

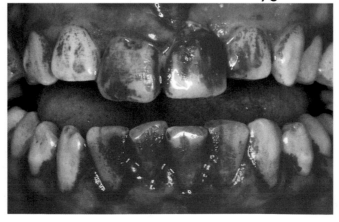

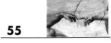

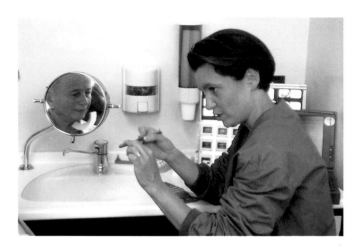

The next step is to show and explain to the patient the requisites and features of a good toothbrush. After deciding on the brushing technique that is most appropriate for the patient's periodontium (see Chapter 3), I begin by explaining how to use the toothbrush, showing the correct technique first on the plastic model and then in the mouth. When deep pockets are present, the periodontium is usually thick; therefore, the Bass technique is the one most frequently taught.

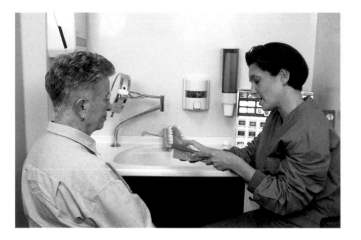

I begin the instruction by telling the patient that:

"The objective is to disrupt the bacteria in the sulcus so that they can no longer release the toxic substances that inflame the gums. To do this you must incline the toothbrush at a 45-degree angle toward the sulcus, as if it were the blade of a knife, so that you feel the tips of the bristles enter the gap. Then, you must move the brush in a very small circular pattern that will enable you to reach and disrupt the bacteria.

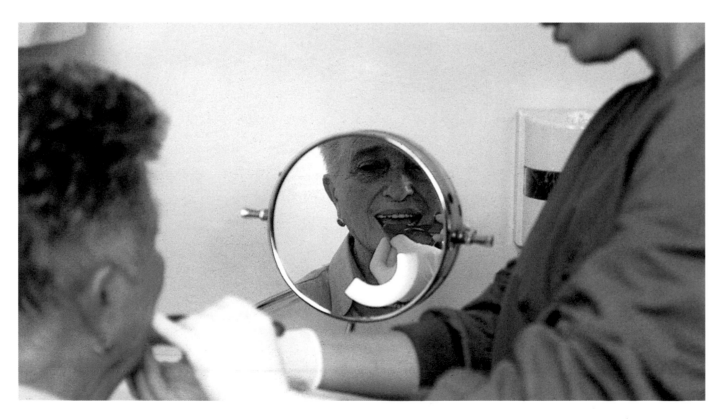

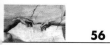

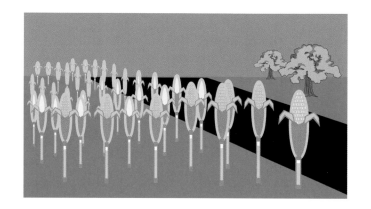

"Think of your mouth as a field of corn cobs! Try to imagine that these accumulations of bacteria are organized like a cob of corn, where each kernel is a bacterium, one beside another and one on top of the other. Therefore, in order to disrupt them it is necessary to separate them from each other, like shelling a cob of corn. Because the bacteria are firmly attached to the surface of the tooth and to one another, disrupting them requires several seconds on each area."

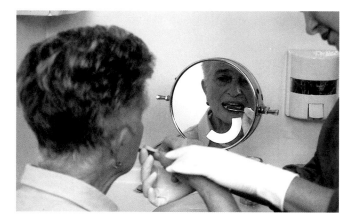

After this, it is advisable to have patients practice the technique in their own mouths to ensure that they have understood. Patients may be shy and reluctant to do it, and in this case I tell them that:

"I have to see if I have explained things adequately!"

The patient usually will not refuse to cooperate.

It is always necessary to ask patients to repeat immediately all the hygiene techniques that have been demonstrated. This makes it possible to achieve a high percentage of memorization.

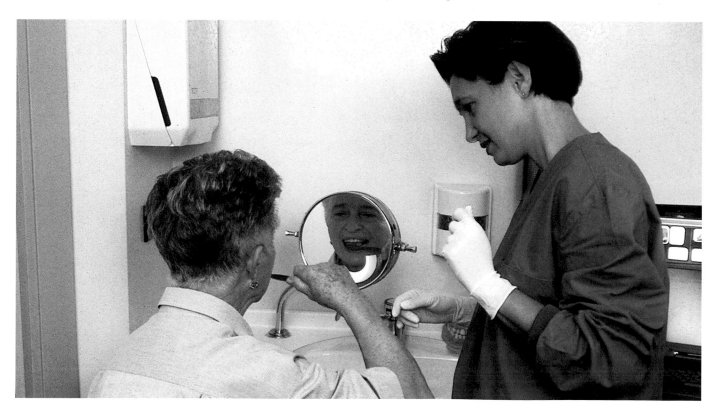

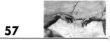

While the patient is practicing, I give some useful advice as to how and when to perform the massage that disrupts the bacterial plaque:

"You may not need to use a mirror. The fundamental thing is to feel the toothbrush between your teeth and your gums. It is very important not to push with the toothbrush because it is the massage and not the pressure that is effective and enables you to remove the bacteria. In fact, if you push too much you risk abrading the gums.

"During the initial period, the gums will bleed while you are brushing, but you must persist, especially in the inflamed areas, because you must remove the bacteria that have caused the bleeding. The mechanical brushing technique will take the place of your body's defense system, which will withdraw because it will no longer be necessary. You will see that the condition of your gums will improve every day until they stop bleeding altogether. You must never see your gums bleeding again!

"It is sufficient to perform this bacteria-disrupting massage once a day. If you consider that you have to reach all areas of your mouth, it is evident that this procedure will require at least 5 or 6 minutes. Initially, when the gums are still bleeding, you will have to stay in the bathroom and rinse the toothbrush, but when there is no longer bleeding you can spend the time, for example, sitting in a comfortable armchair, watching a good film, listening to music, or reading a book. This way, time will pass more quickly! Do this massage at the most convenient and relaxing moment of the day, which is usually the evening.

"Toothpaste is not necessary while you are disrupting the bacteria. Keeping it in your mouth for 5 or 6 minutes could be very annoying and you would not be able to sit comfortably in an armchair because of the lather that forms and the frequent rinses required. Moreover, toothpaste has an abrasive component that might cause problems if it remains in contact with the surface of your teeth too long. I advise you to brush your teeth with toothpaste only after you have completed the massage. This serves to clean and polish them and, above all, to release active substances, such as fluoride, that are useful in fighting caries. In this case, however, the toothbrush must be rotated with a vertical movement from the gum to the tooth. The movement will be downward when you are cleaning the upper teeth and upward when you are cleaning the lower teeth, as if you were cleaning a comb. Then you have to brush the chewing surfaces with an energetic horizontal movement. You may also brush your teeth rapidly, with a toothbrush and toothpaste, after breakfast and lunch to remove any residue of food and to benefit from the protective action of the fluoride."

Many clinicians teach the modified Bass technique, which calls for a circular massage followed immediately by a vertical rotary movement from the gingiva to the tooth. I prefer to separate the two procedures because at recalls I notice that patients only remember the vertical movement and no longer perform the Bass technique. This happens because it is easy for the patient to remember the concept of cleaning the tooth surfaces but not necessarily how to clean the margin of the gingiva. Thus, in the presence of a thick periodontium, the Bass technique has proven to be the most effective for the removal of the plaque along the margin of the gingiva.[7]

In cases in which the periodontium is thick, I try to make patients aware of the fact that they must remember to clean certain areas with particular attention.

"If you carefully observe the margin of your gums, you will notice that they are not on the same level as the surface of your teeth. Therefore, if you limit yourself just to brushing vertically, you will miss the area where the gums and teeth meet. This is the very place that you need to clean well."

Why don't I start working in the patient's mouth during the first appointment? It is useful to determine how much the inflammation will be reduced by the patient's self-performed oral hygiene. Patients must be convinced that their efforts will reduce the bleeding of the gingiva.

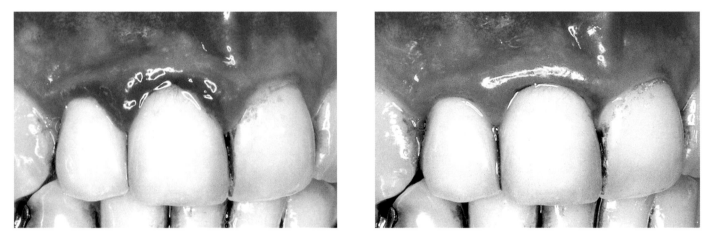

This verification increases both my credibility as a hygienist and the patient's motivation. Patients will gain faith in themselves and will begin to understand that they can really do something for their own teeth and gingiva.

Some patients find it strange that their first appointment is only a "chat" with the hygienist. If this is the case I explain that:

"I don't begin to clean during the first appointment because your gums will be less inflamed after your work at home. Then, during the second appointment, there will be less bleeding and you will feel less discomfort while I clean the pockets."

Naturally, I do not tell patients that this approach serves not only to improve the condition of the tissue, but also to give them confidence in themselves.

Supragingival calculus must be removed during the first appointment only in exceptional cases, that is, when there is a "wall" of calculus. This is also the case when the patient lives far away; a longer appointment may be planned so that it is possible to begin scaling.

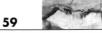
When I follow this procedure and the patient later returns for the second appointment with a noticeable improvement in the condition of the gingiva, the patient is immediately ready to tell me that the merit is mine because I began to clean during the first sitting. This is not the result that I want to obtain! The patient should realize that self-performed oral hygiene has helped to bring about this improvement.

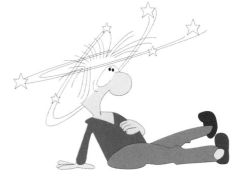

I don't think it is advisable to give the patient any instruments other than a toothbrush during the first sitting. Everything can't be learned at once! Only during the next hygiene appointments, in which I perform scaling, do I teach the patient how to use an appropriate interdental instrument and eventually other adjunctive aids that may be necessary to complete oral hygiene.

When the appointment terminates, I remind patients that they can do a great deal to help themselves:

"We have finished for today. In the next few days, concentrate on this brushing technique and you will notice an improvement in your gums. Later you will also have to use an instrument that will enable you to clean between your teeth, where the toothbrush cannot reach. But we will talk about that the next time."

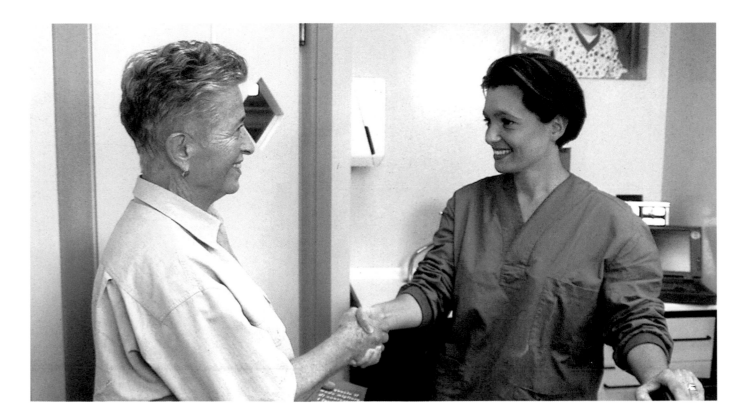

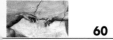

Our conversation terminates in this manner, and patients leave, satisfied with what has been explained, but above all curious to find out if what they have been told will prove to be true: The brushing technique alone can reduce the bleeding of the gingiva!

At the end of the first appointment, I record the patient's personal information in the hygiene chart (any particular episode, an important event, a sad occasion, an illness that may affect a member of the family, etc) so that during the following appointments a short glance at these notes will be enough to remind me of our previous conversation. Frequently, however, the relationship that has been established is so friendly that it is not necessary to consult these annotations.

When patients arrive for the second appointment, I ask them for the first time to sit in the dentist's chair. They are usually anxious to tell me that the brushing technique is working. I have noticed that patients find it more relaxing to chat for a few minutes before I begin treatment, so I try to exchange a few words with them while I am putting on the necessary precautionary garments. This approach gives me the opportunity to greet patients cordially and avoids the shock of finding me dressed like a surgeon who is ready to operate. The patient has learned to have faith in me, and, despite the fact that I now appear hardly recognizable, they are willing to undergo the treatment that I explained in the previous appointment.

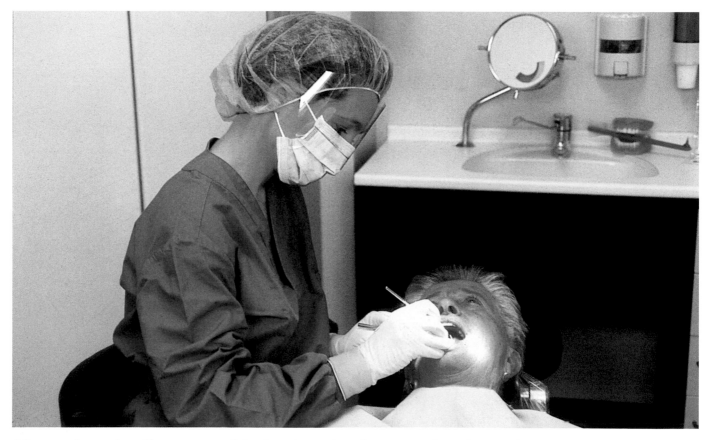

After verifying the effectiveness of the brushing that the patient has done at home…

…I sometimes find that the use of a single-tufted toothbrush is necessary and must be included in the patient's home care.

First, I describe the characteristics of the instrument, and I demonstrate its use in the patient's oral cavity…

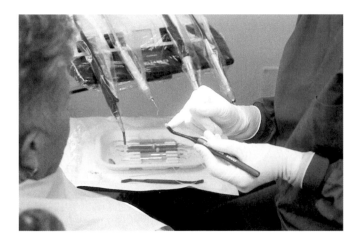 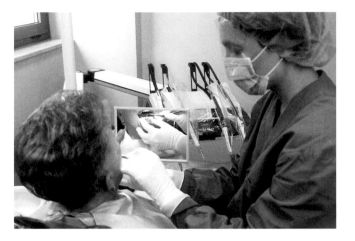

… then I ask the patient to practice its use in my presence.

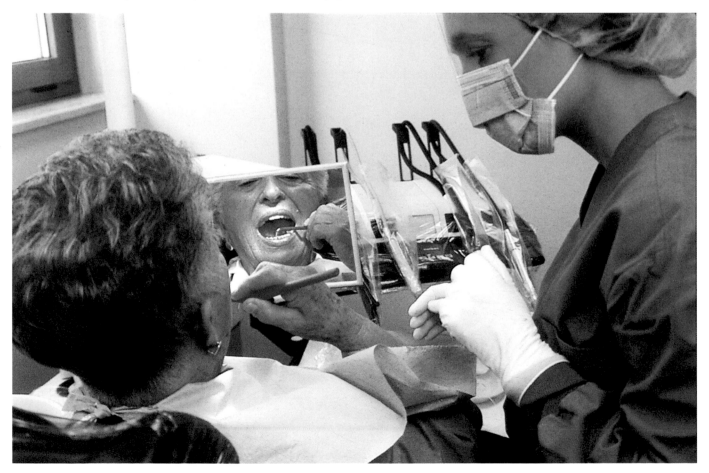

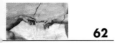

As for interdental instruments, it may be necessary to teach patients to use dental floss.

I explain how to wind it around the fingers, and then I insert it in the patients' interdental spaces, standing behind them as if my hands were theirs.

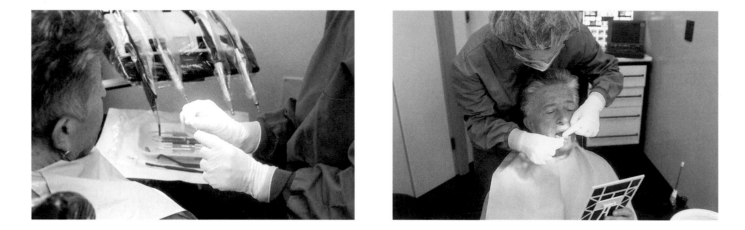

When this demonstration terminates, I ask the patient to practice so that I can verify that this technique is being performed correctly.

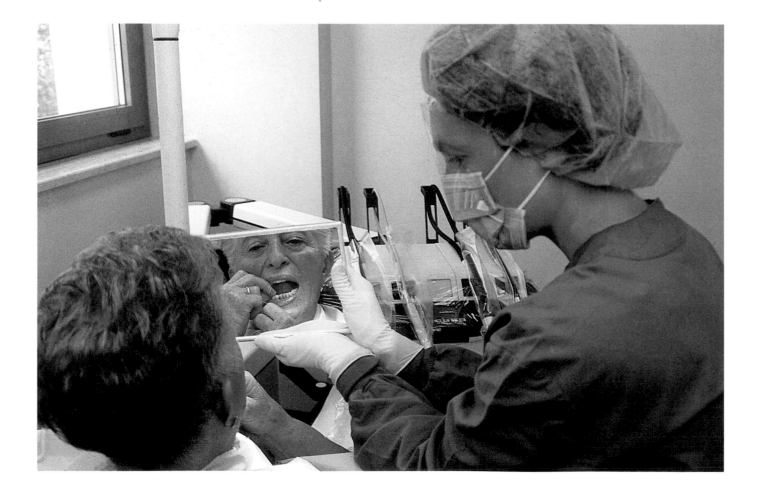

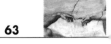
The use of an interproximal brush may be required. If so, a choice is made between the type to be inserted in a handle...

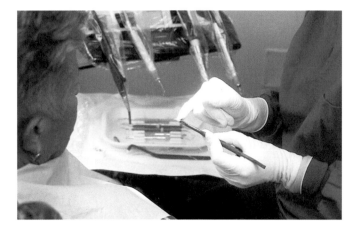 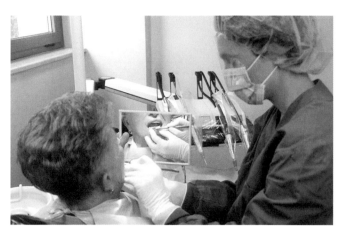

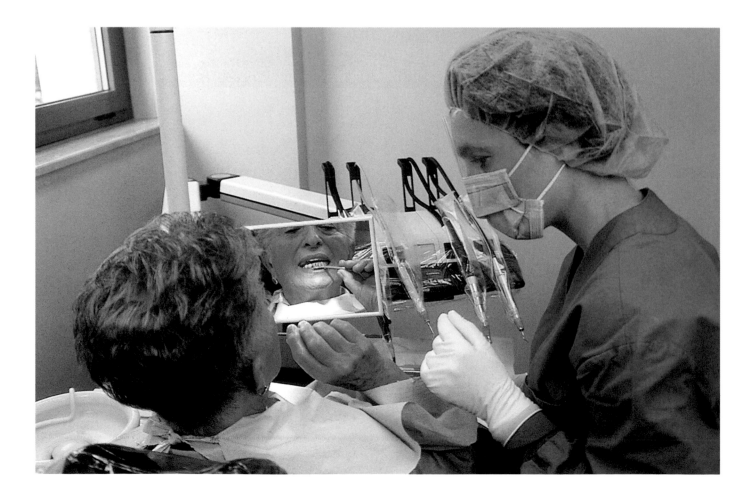

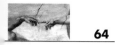

…and a longer one with a metal core that can take the place of a handle.

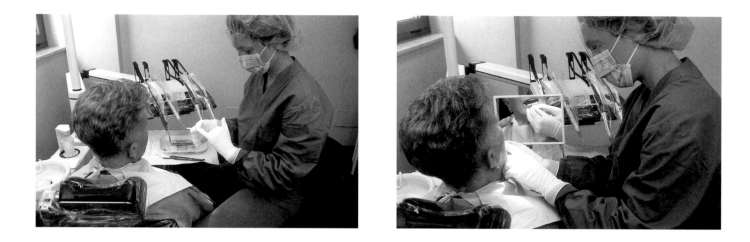

You should realize that the patient is not accustomed to cleaning interdental spaces; therefore, more careful attention must be given to these often neglected areas that are more easily affected by periodontal disease.

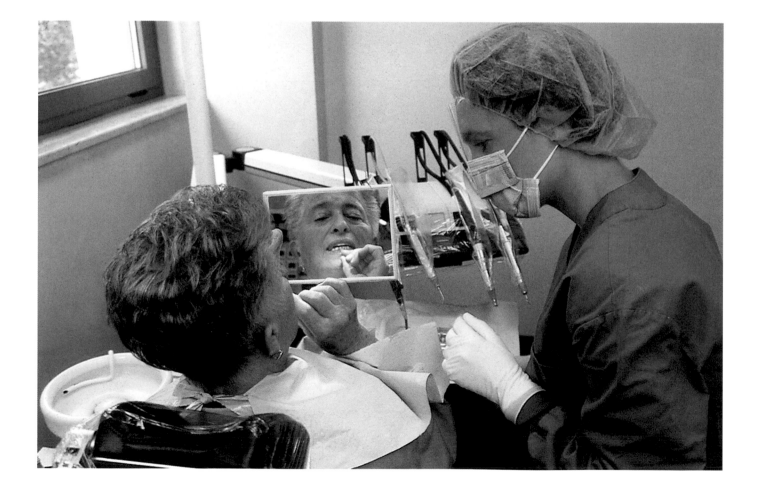

Sometimes the patient may not be able to find the suggested instruments on the market and consequently will not be able to perform effective home care. We risk losing precious time! In order to avoid this inconvenience, the dental office should arrange to supply the patient with all of the required hygiene instruments.

Each time patients come for an appointment, I renew my discourse about the importance of their collaboration[1] to refresh their awareness of the problem and to keep them adequately informed. This is, of course, if patients are interested in saving their teeth. Most patients want to save their teeth, and the task of the dental hygienist is to help them.

Often, the chewing function of the patient with reduced periodontal support is compromised in such a way that it is necessary to resort to a prosthetic rehabilitation; a fixed type is generally used, which often means that implants will have to be placed. The patient who has both natural teeth and implants must be motivated in exactly the same way as the patient who has a natural dentition.

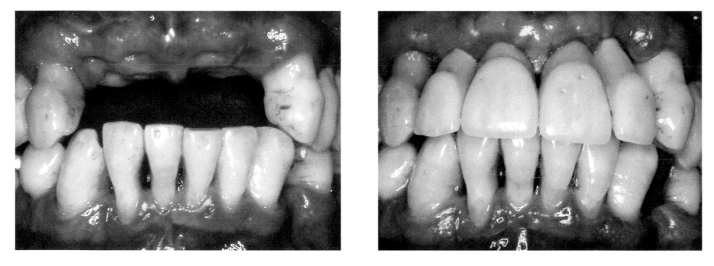

One of the most serious concerns that torments patients who have to undergo implant surgery is the fear of "rejection," but I try to reassure them by explaining that:

"There is a high percentage of success with implants. However, you must be aware that plaque may also colonize around the implant, just as it does around the tooth. If this plaque is not removed adequately, it will accumulate and could eventually cause the loss of the implant itself. Therefore, like teeth, implants must be kept clean; otherwise, you will lose them, just as you have already lost some of your teeth. However, we do not have to face this problem now. When the times comes, I will teach you how to clean implants effectively.

From the start of treatment, the patient must be motivated to carry out a proper program of oral hygiene around the implant, even if it has not yet been placed in the oral cavity.

I supply instructions regarding peri-implant oral hygiene according to the implant technique chosen by the dentist. Today, there is a tendency to divide implant techniques into two categories: submerged (two-stage) implants and nonsubmerged (one-stage) implants.

In the submerged technique (a), the implants remain buried under the oral mucosa for a few months until the moment of abutment connection. During this period, procedures of hygiene are not required, but mouthrinses with an antiseptic solution should be performed until the wound heals. The surface of the implant, generally the healing screw, may, however, be exposed to the oral cavity because of a fenestration in the oral mucosa (b). Plaque will then accumulate on the surfaces of these implants; therefore, it must be removed. In this case, I give the patient instructions regarding the appropriate techniques (see Chapter 3).

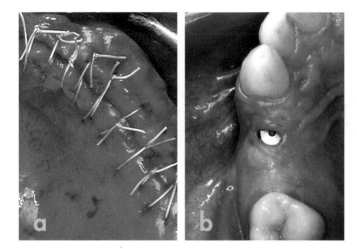

In the nonsubmerged technique (c), or at the moment of abutment connection if the submerged technique is preferred (d), the implant will be permanently exposed to the oral cavity. Therefore, it is necessary to demonstrate the correct procedures to keep it clean (see Chapter 3).

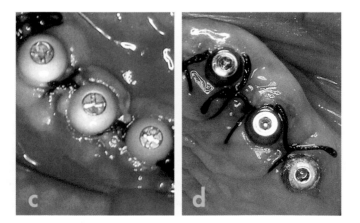

After the prosthesis has been applied, I teach the patient the techniques required to clean its surfaces properly.

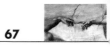
Even when dealing with edentulous patients who decide to undergo implant surgery, it is necessary to explain from the start how important their collaboration is for the success of the treatment.

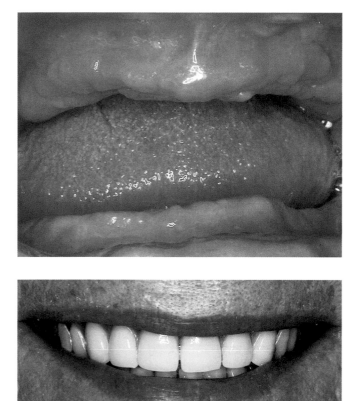

It is not, however, difficult to motivate edentulous patients who have lost their teeth little by little, and who come to the dentist's office specifically requesting implants and are willing to spend a lot of time and money. These patients know exactly what will happen if they do not take care of their teeth, and they have learned to fear the consequences that may occur because of neglect.

After the prosthesis has been inserted, I teach the patient the proper techniques to maintain an adequate hygiene status around the implants. These techniques are similar to those used in cleaning natural teeth (see Chapter 3).

As when dealing with natural teeth, I remind the patient of the important role that self-performed oral hygiene has in maintaining the results of the treatment:

"Your collaboration is essential for the maintenance of these implants. We have done everything possible to improve your situation, but now you must keep the implants that support this prosthesis in good condition. The dentist has designed the prosthesis so that it can be cleaned easily and you will have no difficulty in removing plaque. If you come for periodic checkups, I will give you advice that will help you reach this goal."

This simulation of an appointment aimed at motivating patients affected by periodontal disease has reproduced the method that I personally use to obtain the patients' collaboration. The content may, of course, be modified, giving less importance to or omitting some parts and amplifying others according to the relevant factors of each case, such as the clinical character of patients' disorders, their knowledge of periodontal disease, their personal backgrounds, and their willingness and ability to cooperate. The style of communication that the hygienist chooses may also vary in relation to these factors.

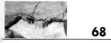

STYLES OF COMMUNICATION

An excellent style of communication is the democratic one, in which we use the resources of both the patient and the hygienist to develop two-way communication. This helps to establish reciprocal trust and induces the patient to participate actively. This is the ideal approach, but it is not always possible to use it; on some occasions, it may be necessary to use other styles of communication that are not ideal but that, in given circumstances, are more appropriate than the democratic one.

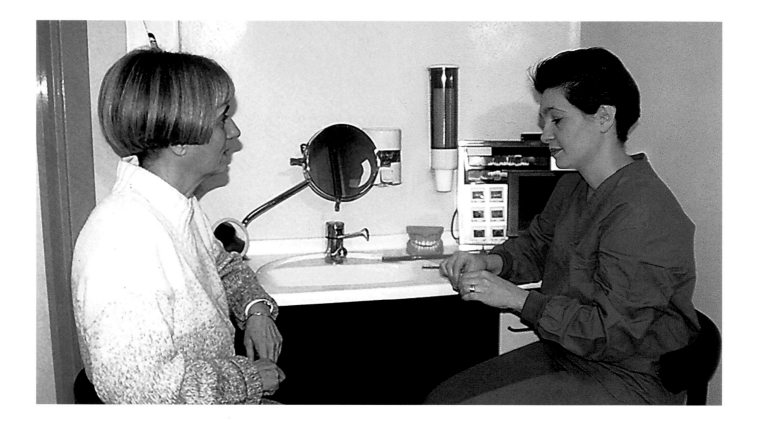

At times we have to be authoritative, trying to obtain cooperation by taking advantage of our professional role. This may occur during maintenance therapy when the patient's efforts have slackened and need to be stimulated and prompted. Our authoritarianism is better accepted in this context because we have already established a friendly relationship with the patient, so we can dare to offer a few incisive instructions.

In other cases, we may momentarily find ourselves being paternal, that is, we may try to protect the patient from the risk being faced because of the patient's negligence. Sometimes we may also be permissive, telling patients that if they do not have the time to brush their teeth, we will put aside that problem until later. These styles of communication, which do not lead to positive results, should, however, be taken into consideration when we are dealing with a patient who is worried about other problems regarding, for example, health or family, that are more important at that moment than the bacteria in the gingival sulcus. In these cases, it is better to postpone to a more suitable moment the democratic approach, which will enable us to reestablish the fundamental collaboration with the patient.

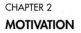

FAILURE OF COMMUNICATION: THE MOST COMMON ERRORS THAT IMPEDE DIALOGUE WITH THE PATIENT

Good communication is essential to prevent patients from assuming a negative attitude or developing a mental block that might induce them to ignore the hygienist's advice. Although it may seem useless, it is important to make every attempt to convince the patient, especially if the patient appears to be reluctant or perplexed even after the warnings and advice that the hygienist has given. Before accepting that it is impossible to motivate a patient, we should ask ourselves if we have done everything in our power to successfully communicate with the person.

Communication may fail for various reasons.

We may have used inappropriate words or terms that are too scientific, or perhaps we have not offered a clear explanation or have taken for granted knowledge that the patient does not have. These errors will all impede adequate communication.

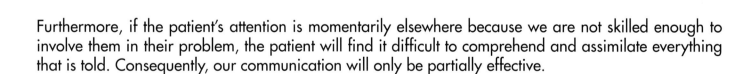

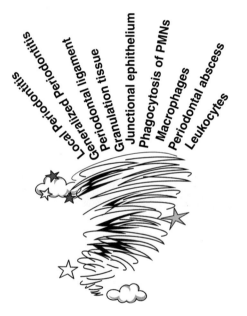

Furthermore, if the patient's attention is momentarily elsewhere because we are not skilled enough to involve them in their problem, the patient will find it difficult to comprehend and assimilate everything that is told. Consequently, our communication will only be partially effective.

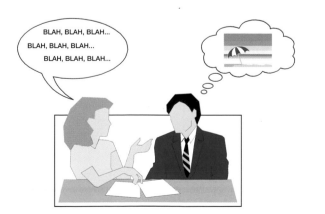

Sometimes we may not be able to alleviate the patient's anxiety, and in some cases, because of differences in culture and lifestyle, we may not succeed in conveying our message. Whatever the problem, the hygienist should always supply the patient with further explanations, utilizing simpler terms that may be able to clarify concepts that were not understood. At the same time, the hygienist's efforts to make the message clear help to establish a mutual understanding between patient and hygienist.

Failure is often temporary because it can lead to positive results if it is carefully analyzed and the outcome of this analysis is used to modify the parts of the motivation that were not effective. Success is not guaranteed at the start of our profession as dental hygienists, but we should make every effort to hit the mark with all potential patients. Experience increases the efficacy of our motivational skills.[5]

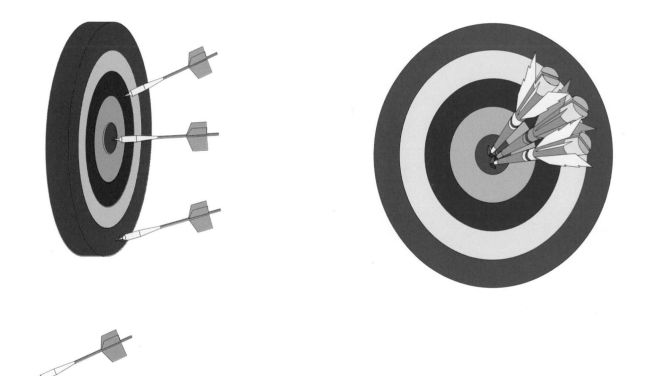

We must attempt to do not only what appears possible, but also what appears impossible if we want to increase our probability of success.

We will be able to verify that our motivation has been effective, not only during active therapy, but also subsequently, observing the assiduity with which the patient complies with periodic recalls (compliance).

REFERENCES

1. Emler BF, Windchy AM, Zaino SW, Feldman SM, Scheetz JP. The value of repetition and reinforcement in improving oral hygiene performance. J Periodontol 1980;51:228–234.

2. Lindhe J, Nyman S. The effect of plaque control and surgical pocket elimination on the establishment and maintenance of periodontal health. A longitudinal study of periodontal treatment in cases of advanced disease. J Clin Periodontol 1975;2:67–79.

3. Lindhe J, Westfelt E, Nyman S, Socransky SS, Heijl L, Bratthall G. Healing following surgical/non-surgical treatment of periodontal disease. J Clin Periodontol 1982;9:115–128.

4. Rosling B, Nyman S, Lindhe J. The effect of systematic plaque control on bone regeneration in infrabony pockets. J Clin Periodontol 1976;3:38–53.

5. Rozencweig D. Manuale di Prevenzione Dentaria, capitoli 3, 4. Milano: Masson, 1990.

6. Stewart JE, Jacobs-Schoen M, Padilla MR, Maeder LA, Wolfe GR, Hartz GW. The effect of a cognitive behavioral intervention on oral hygiene. J Clin Periodontol 1991;18:219–222.

7. Waerhaug J. Effect of toothbrushing on subgingival plaque formation. J Periodontol 1981;52:30–34.

**EXPERIENCE
IS THE BEST TEACHER**

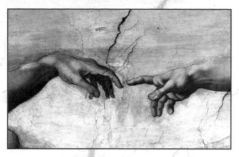

CHAPTER 3

**PLAQUE CONTROL
AT TEETH AND IMPLANTS**

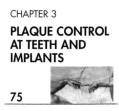
The patient's self-performed oral hygiene (plaque control) is a mainstay in the prevention of periodontal disease. In fact, without the patient's constant collaboration, the periodontal treatments performed by professional operators have little success and, above all, the results obtained are not long lasting.

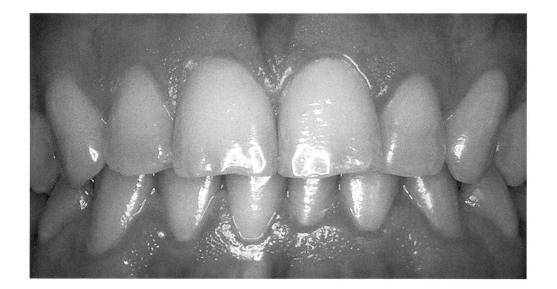

After assessing the condition of the patient's oral cavity, the hygienist must demonstrate the correct oral hygiene procedures, suggesting the appropriate instruments and techniques. Oral hygiene must be monitored during periodontal therapy and, if necessary, the initial program must be modified to improve the status of hygiene and maintain the health of the oral cavity. There are many instruments for oral hygiene at the hygienist's disposal, and the market also offers a wide selection of products for self-performed oral hygiene. In the course of my work as a hygienist, I have made definite choices regarding products and techniques that have satisfied me and that enable me to reach my objectives.

In this chapter, I will explain my preferences with regard to:

- Plaque-disclosing agents
- Toothbrushes
- Toothbrushing techniques
- Toothpastes
- Interdental instruments
- Special cleaning devices

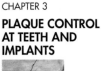
▶ **PLAQUE-DISCLOSING AGENTS**

The function of plaque-disclosing agents is to stain and therefore reveal the presence of bacterial plaque that has accumulated on tooth surfaces.[21,29] This staining enables the patient to visualize their own plaque and thereby to improve the efficacy of their efforts to remove it.

Plaque-disclosing agents are available in different forms: solutions that may be applied to teeth, tablets (eg, Red-Cote, Butler, Chicago, IL; Plaque Finder, Pro-Dentec, Batesville, AR; Dis-Plaque, Oral-B, Boston, MA), or wafers saturated with a disclosing solution (eg, Rondell Red, SDI, Sweden; ESRO Plak, Paro, Switzerland).

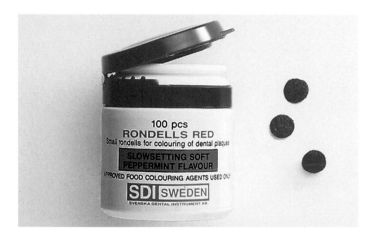

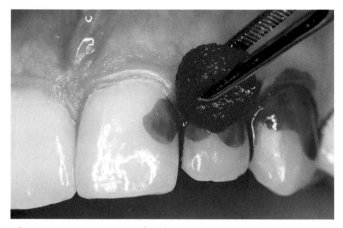

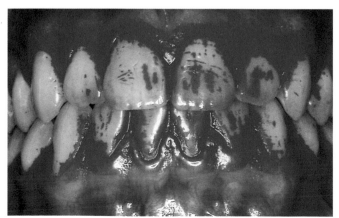

The most common disclosing agents are generally composed of a fuchsia-colored erythrosine sodium solution.

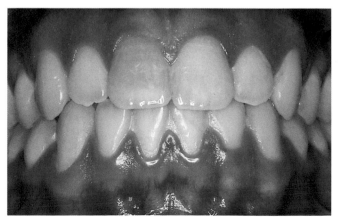

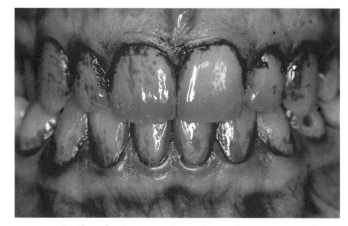

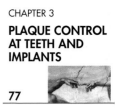
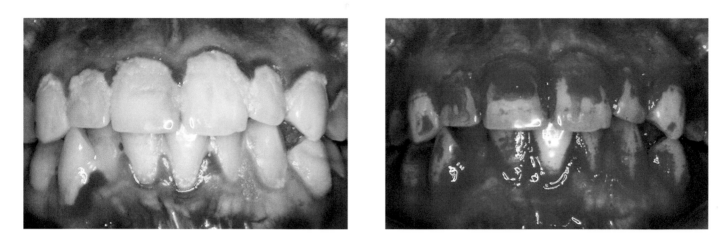

However, two-tone agents, such as violet stain, which contains methylene blue and erythrosin, are also available on the market. This solution makes it possible to distinguish an old plaque accumulation from a more recent one by means of the more intense or less intense stain that results when the product is applied to teeth.

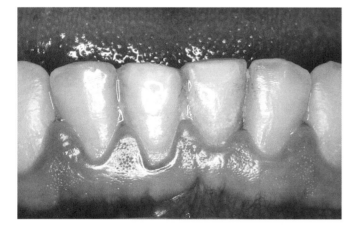
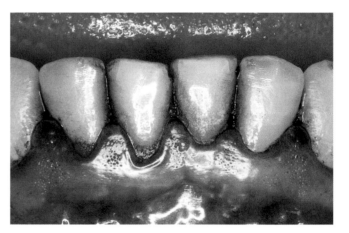

After carefully observing the areas where plaque has been evidenced, the patient can then remove the deposits from the dental surfaces with adequate brushing.

One disadvantage of disclosing agents is that they leave the mucosa stained for some time, and this may create an esthetic problem for some patients. As for lips, this inconvenience may be eliminated by protecting them with petroleum jelly, while the staining of the tongue can be reduced by utilizing saturated wafers, which enable the operator to apply the product to teeth with more precision.

The patient may use the disclosing agent before performing the mechanical techniques to visualize the plaque and learn the use of the recommended instruments, or it may be applied after self-performed oral hygiene to identify sites at which the mechanical techniques have been inadequate, thus enabling an evaluation of the efficacy of the patient's own efforts. Naturally, once the patient has learned to use the suggested instruments well, plaque-disclosing agents will no longer need to be applied during self-performed oral hygiene.

During periodontal treatment, the hygienist may use the plaque-disclosing agents to evaluate the patient's technical ability.

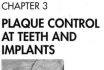
TOOTHBRUSHES

The toothbrush is an indispensable instrument for the removal of plaque and food debris from dental surfaces, but it does not enable the patient to achieve complete interdental hygiene,[8,12] which requires the use of a more appropriate instrument (see the section on interdental instruments).

There are many types of toothbrushes that differ in size, form, stiffness of bristles, and length and array of tufts. Although the "ideal" toothbrush does not exist, various studies have demonstrated the greater efficacy of a manual toothbrush with a short head and synthetic bristles with rounded ends.[9, 29]

SHORT HEAD

The short head has fewer tufts and is considered functional because it can easily reach all areas of the mouth. In fact, the fewer tufts present on the head of the toothbrush, the more effective it will be in removing plaque.[7]

One example of a toothbrush with a short head is the Butler Gum 409 Compact,

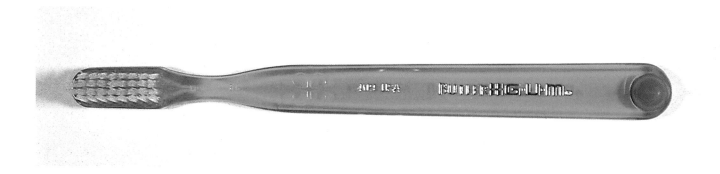

which is shorter than the 411 because it has two fewer rows of tufts.

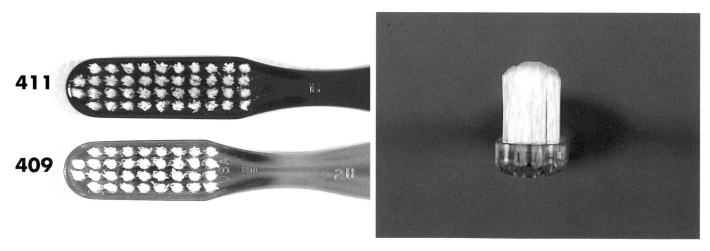

411

409

In addition, the two central rows of tufts are longer than the lateral ones.

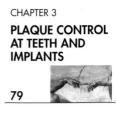

Other examples are the Oral-B Restage Indicator P30 and P35 toothbrushes, which are shorter than the P40. In this type of toothbrush, the four rows of tufts are all the same length, and the central ones indicate the degree of wear.

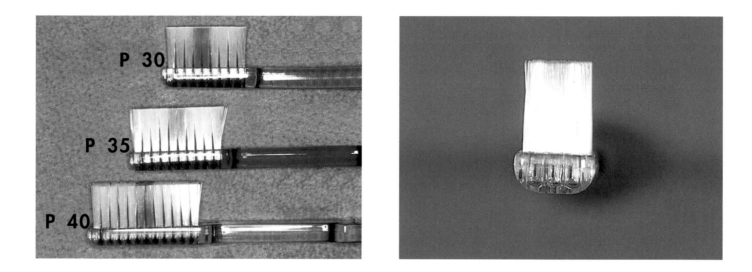

There are no substantial differences between the two types of toothbrushes with regard to their efficacy in the removal of plaque. The choice is subjective. Some patients prefer toothbrushes that are rather stiff, while others prefer softer ones.

SYNTHETIC BRISTLES

Synthetic bristles (eg, nylon, tynes) are the best choice because they do not absorb water and therefore remain stiff, whereas natural ones tend to lose their original consistency and become very soft and therefore ineffective in removing plaque.[7]

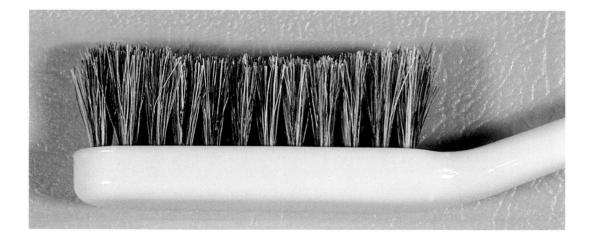

From "Atlante di Odontoiatria" directed by K.H. Rateitschak - N. 4 Carioprofilassi e Terapia Conservativa - Peter Raithe in collaboration with Gunther Rau - Piccin Nuova Libraria s.p.a. PADOVA.

Furthermore, natural bristles, unlike synthetic ones, contain gaps in which bacteria can colonize, and they do not have rounded ends, which is a very important feature.

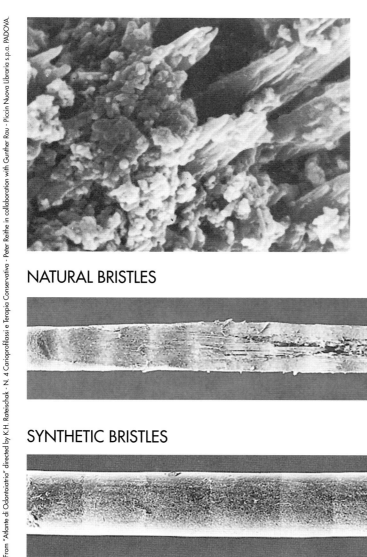

NATURAL BRISTLES

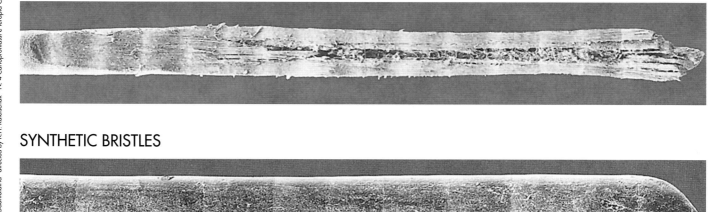

SYNTHETIC BRISTLES

ROUNDED ENDS

Rounded ends are indispensable because they reduce lesions of the gingiva. Toothbrushes with sharp bristles have a more abrasive effect on the gingival tissue than those with round-ended bristles.[1,10]

The longer a toothbrush is used, the more its signs of wear increase, and consequently its cleaning potential diminishes.[14] Due consideration should also be given to other factors that determine the wear of the toothbrush, such as the length and frequency of brushing, the brushing force applied, and the quality of the toothpaste. These factors vary a great deal according to the individual, and any variations will determine the rapidity with which the toothbrush begins to show signs of wear. Therefore, the toothbrush must be replaced when it loses its initial form and becomes deformed and matted.

As a general rule, it is not advisable to use the same toothbrush for more than about 2.5 months. In this length of time, the formation of the bristle ends changes, and this alteration reduces the potential of the toothbrush to eliminate plaque.[18,26]

TOOTHBRUSHING TECHNIQUES

Different toothbrushing techniques can be classified in relation to the type of movement that the toothbrush performs.[21]

Whichever technique is used, it is important that it not damage teeth and gums. In fact, improper toothbrushing may traumatize the gingiva and provoke a recession if the incorrect procedure is continued. Cementum and dentin may be more exposed because of this gingival recession and may therefore be more subject to abrasion at the neck caused by toothpaste.[30]

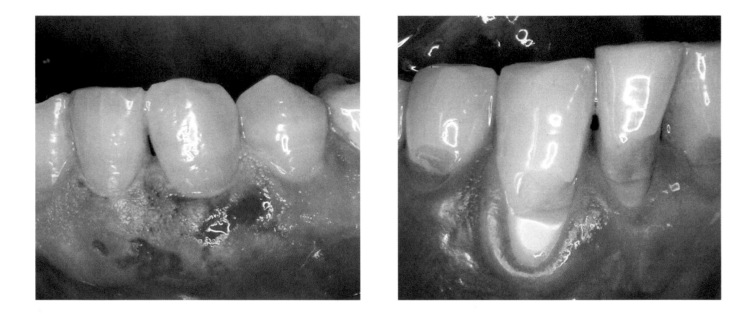

Even an excessive brushing force, especially in the horizontal direction, may cause diffused dental abrasions.[1]

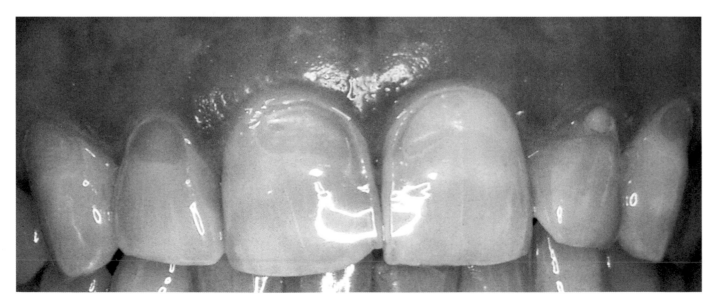

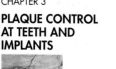
Therefore, possible damage to the gingiva and the hard tissue of teeth may be due to:

- **The ends of the bristles**
- **The direction of brushing**
- **The abrasiveness of the toothpaste**
- **The brushing force applied**

Initially, whichever brushing technique is used, it is preferable to use a dry toothbrush with no toothpaste to enable the bristles to adequately disrupt the bacteria. When the first phase has been completed, the toothbrush will then be used with toothpaste.

Several authors[6,11,31] have devised brushing techniques, but it is difficult to determine which is actually the most effective. Various problems may arise in the cleaning of a patient's oral cavity, depending on the anatomic structure of the individual's periodontium. I have found that the Bass technique and the vertical rotary technique are able to resolve these problems satisfactorily.[29]

▷ BASS TECHNIQUE

The head of the toothbrush is inclined at a 45-degree angle to the gingival margin so that the ends of the bristles penetrate into the gingival sulcus.

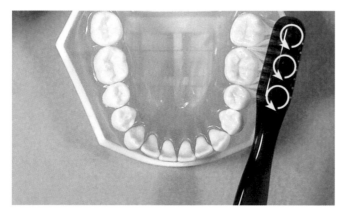

Then, with light pressure, short back-and-forth vibratory movements are effected with the toothbrush, maintaining the ends of the bristles in the sulcus.[6] Experience has taught me to prefer a vibratory-circular movement instead of the back-and-forth stroke to prevent the patient from effecting long horizontal movements, which can cause gingival and dental lesions.

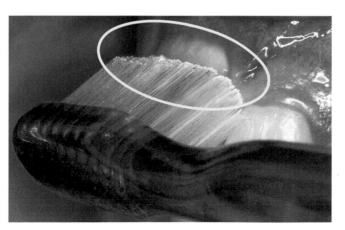

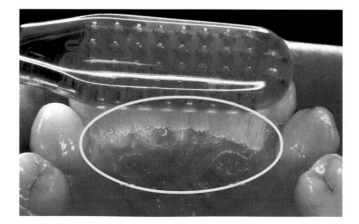

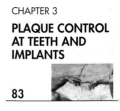
The Bass technique enables the toothbrush to disrupt the bacteria that have accumulated both above and below the gingival margin because the bristles penetrate as far as 0.9 mm beneath this margin. This helps to prevent the formation of subgingival plaque.[32]

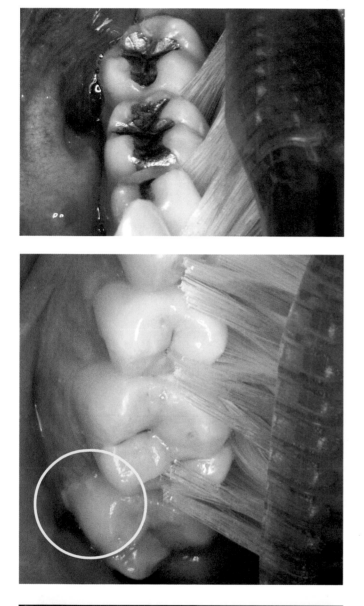

The procedure necessary to disrupt the plaque on all tooth surfaces requires about 4 or 5 minutes, and it is sufficient to perform this thorough cleaning once a day.[20] If the patient decides to effect this thorough cleaning before going to bed, after each meal a rapid brushing will be sufficient to remove any food debris.

Despite the use of a short-headed toothbrush, it is sometimes difficult to brush the surface of the posterior teeth adequately; therefore, it will be necessary to recommend another instrument to clean these specific areas (see the section on special cleaning devices).

When cleaning the lingual surfaces of the anterior teeth in cases in which the dental arch limits the correct horizontal positioning of the toothbrush, the latter may be positioned vertically, inserting the tufts that are closest to the handle into the sulcus to obtain proper access along the margin of the gingiva.

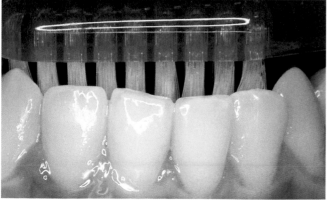

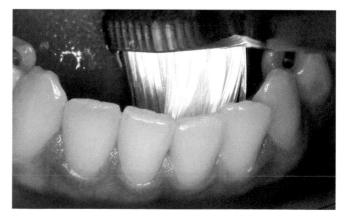

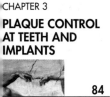
The Bass technique has proven to be particularly effective when the anatomic structure of the patient presents a thick periodontium in which the gingival surface is not on the same level as the tooth surface.

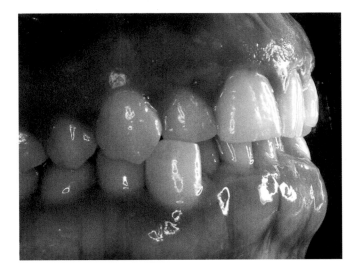

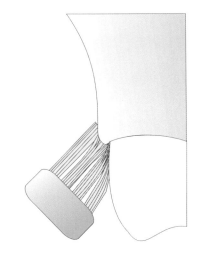

Therefore, this technique may be effective in the following cases:

1. When the gingivae are healthy

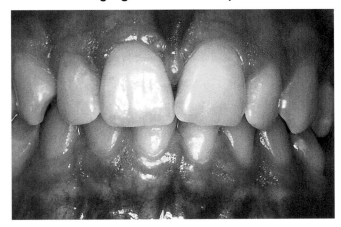

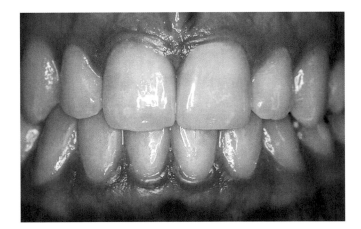

2. In the presence of gingivitis or periodontal disease

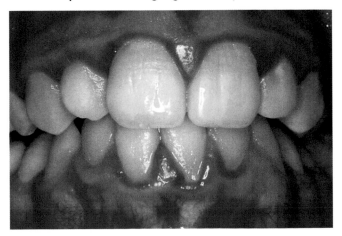

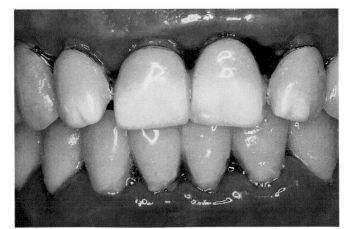

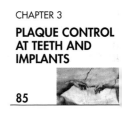

3. Around the peri-implant mucosa

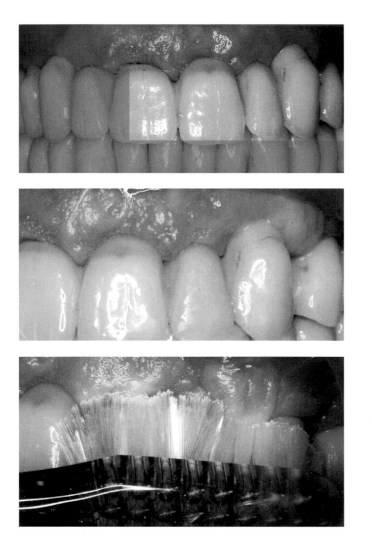

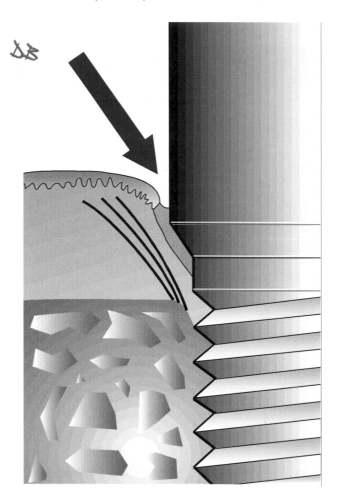

The Bass technique is used to disrupt adequately plaque that has accumulated between the peri-implant mucosa and the Toronto prosthesis. A toothbrush with two rows of tufts is utilized because it enables the patient to obtain proper access between the margin of the mucosa and the prosthesis.

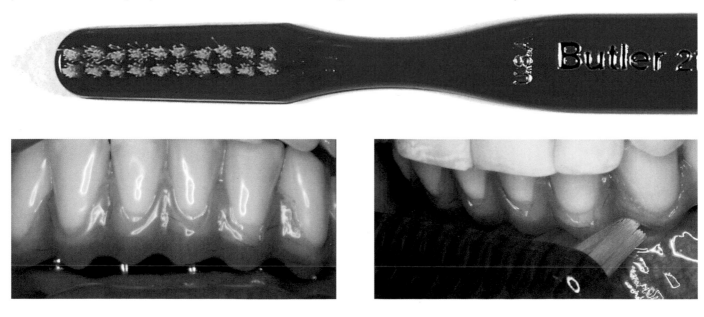

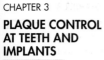
It is also possible to use the Bass technique in the presence of fixed orthodontic appliances, utilizing a toothbrush with two rows of tufts, which facilitates proper access between the gingival margin and the brackets.

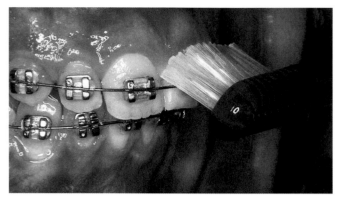 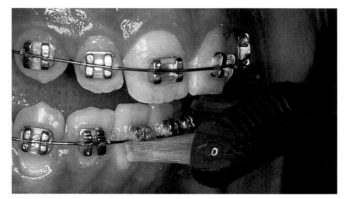

▷ MODIFIED BASS TECHNIQUE

The first phase of this technique is identical to the Bass technique.

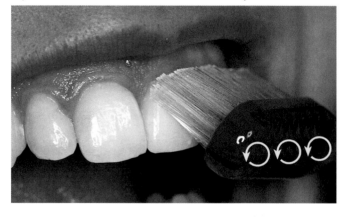

The modified technique calls for the head of the toothbrush to be rotated toward the occlusal surface of the teeth after the vibratory movement in the gingival sulcus has been completed.

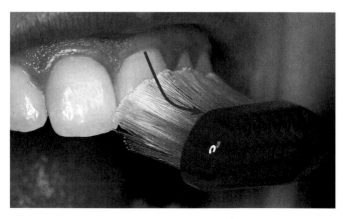

Clinical experience has taught me not to suggest this modification because I have noticed that, in general, patients easily forget the vibratory movement and only perform the rotation toward the occlusal surface of the tooth, thus skipping the gingival margin, which should never be neglected.

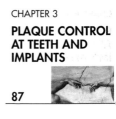
▷ **VERTICAL ROTARY TECHNIQUE**

The bristles of the toothbrush are positioned on the gingiva, and then the toothbrush head is slowly rotated in the occlusal direction, ie, from the gingiva toward the tooth.[29]

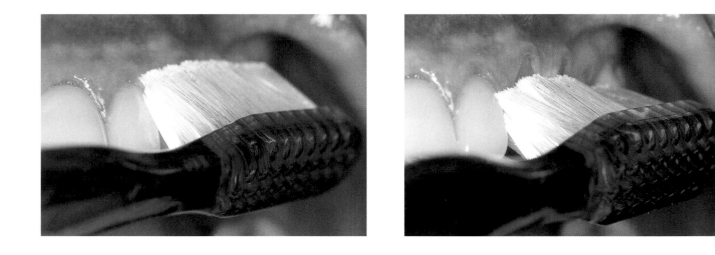

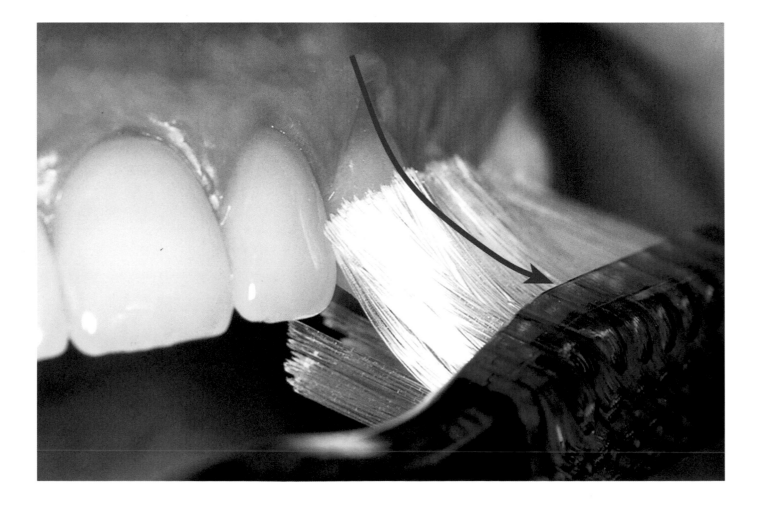

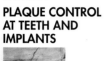
This technique is appropriate for patients with a thin periodontium, who have a predisposition for gingival recessions. It is also suitable where gingival recessions are already present and the surface of the gingiva is on the same level as the tooth surface. Thus, it is easy to remove the plaque along the gingival margin using the vertical rotary movement alone.

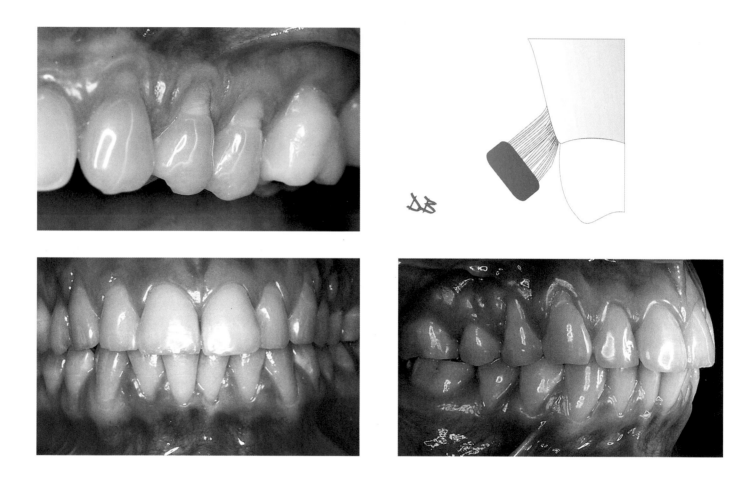

The same technique may be used on both the buccal and the lingual surfaces of the Toronto prosthesis at implants. It is not suitable for cleaning abutments.

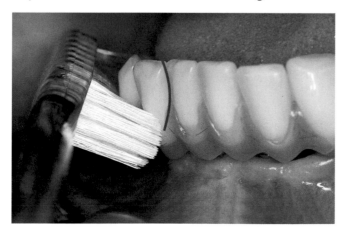

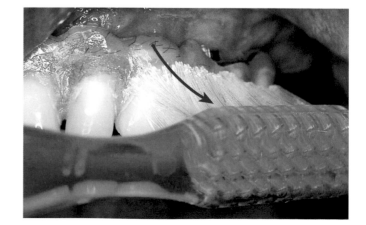

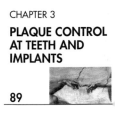
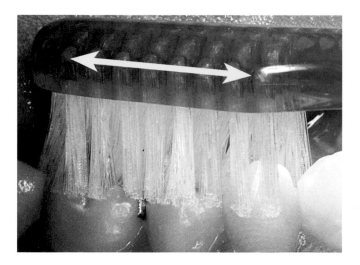

Whichever technique is chosen, the occlusal surfaces are cleaned using a horizontal brushing technique, moving the toothbrush in an anteroposterior direction.

TOOTHPASTES

After careful daily brushing performed with a dry toothbrush, and also during brushing after each meal, it is advisable to use toothpaste to polish teeth and to clean, refresh, and deodorize the oral cavity. Toothpastes make it possible to deliver some active agents to the tooth surfaces for preventive and therapeutic purposes. I suggest that toothpaste be applied with a toothbrush, effecting a vertical-rotary movement in the occlusal direction, starting from the gingiva.

Toothpastes contain various ingredients, and each of these components has its own function.

- Abrasive substances (eg, silica, alumina, calcium phosphate, calcium carbonate) polish the tooth surfaces, but they can also scratch them to the extent that it is possible to find lesions on the teeth caused by an excessively abrasive toothpaste. The abrasive effect should clean adequately without scratching.

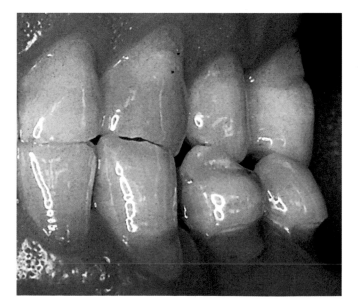

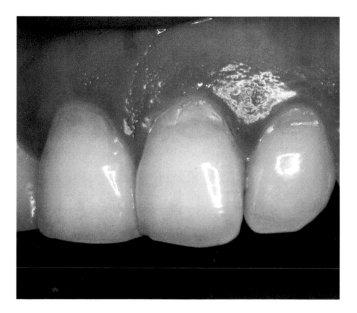

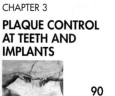
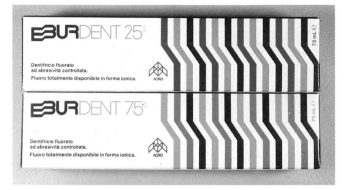

Some toothpastes, among them Eburdent (Beta-farma, Italy), Elmex (GABA International, Germany), and Bioclin (Laboratoires Ganassini, France), declare their degree of abrasiveness, that is, the relative dentin abrasion (RDA). A low RDA is indicated when the patient has implants or presents signs of dental hypersensitivity, gingival recession, and/or enamel abrasions.

- Detergents give the product its foaminess and reinforce the action of the abrasives. The detergent most commonly used is sodium lauryl sulphate.

- Thickeners and emollients, such as glycerin and silicates, prevent the toothpaste from drying out.

- Sweeteners, such as xylitol and sorbitol, sweeten the toothpaste.

- Flavorings, such as menthol or aromatic substances with a fruit flavor, make toothpaste more refreshing and pleasant to use.

- Active ingredients, such as fluoride, antiseptics, desensitizers, and other substances, are delivered to the tooth surfaces through toothpastes, which are an excellent vehicle.

Toothpastes that contain fluorides, especially sodium fluoride, are extremely useful in the prevention of caries.

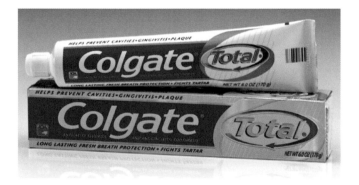

In recent years, triclosan has been introduced into toothpastes; this ingredient, combined with zinc citrate (eg, Mentadent-P, Cheesebrough-Ponds) or with a copolymer (eg, Colgate Total, Colgate-Palmolive), is effective in reducing plaque and gingivitis.[22]

In fact, triclosan not only has antiseptic properties, but also antiphlogistic effects.[3,4,17]

It is difficult to combine chlorhexidine into the formula of toothpastes because it interacts with the sodium lauryl sulphate, reducing the potential of chlorhexidine to inhibit the formation of plaque.[5]

Toothpastes that contain desensitizers, such as potassium nitrate (eg, Emoform-Actisens, Byk Gulden, Germany) or potassium oxalate (eg, Protect, Butler), have a moderate potential to close the dentinal tubules, thus limiting the rapid movements of fluid inside the tubules that cause sensations of pain (see Chapter 6).

Toothpastes that contain pyrophosphates (eg, Colgate Tartar Control, Colgate-Palmolive, New York, NY) can reduce the formation of supragingival calculus.[23]

▶ INTERDENTAL INSTRUMENTS

The interdental spaces cannot be properly reached with a toothbrush.[8,12] Other instruments therefore have to be used for interproximal plaque removal and the most suitable adjunctive devices must be selected for each patient.
The choice depends principally on the width of the interdental spaces.[29]

- Dental floss or tape *(a)* is used for interdental spaces that are completely filled by the gingival papillae or in cases in which teeth are crowded and the spaces are therefore very narrow.

- Wooden toothpicks *(b)* are used for interdental spaces that are slightly open.

- Interdental brushes *(c)* are used for interdental spaces that are wide.

From LIFE ART, 1998. Reproduced with permission of Lippincott/Williams & Wilkins.

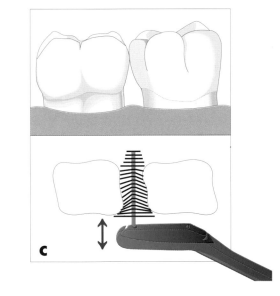

▷ DENTAL FLOSS

Dental floss is composed of numerous nylon filaments that are twisted together and sometimes covered with a thin coat of wax (eg, Butler, Oral-B).

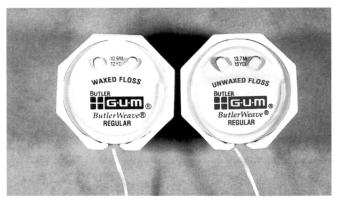

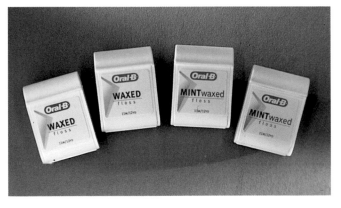

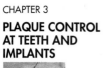
To date, comparison of waxed and unwaxed floss has not evidenced differences in the cleaning potential of either type.[16,19] Findings have shown, however, that waxed floss slides better and can be useful in narrow interproximal spaces.

Tape is a flat monofilament (eg, Glide, W.L. Gore, Flagstaff, AZ), an expanded polytetrafluoro-ethylene (e-PTFE) expanse with a thin wax coating. It is very useful and easy to use when the interdental spaces are very narrow.

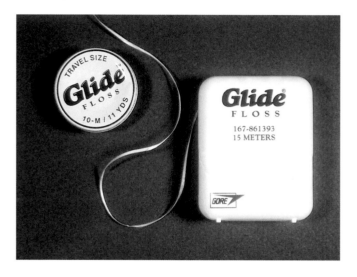

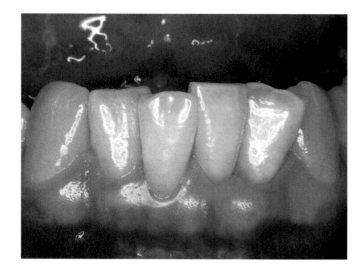

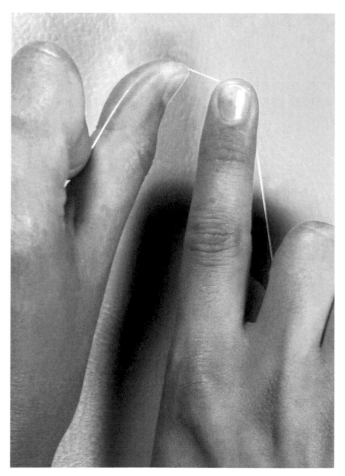

Whichever type is selected, the floss is wound around the middle finger of each hand, keeping a short segment on one side and the remaining longer portion on the other.

When floss is used between the anterior teeth, it is kept taught between the thumb of one hand and the index finger of the other.

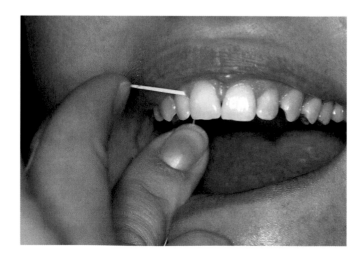

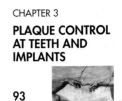
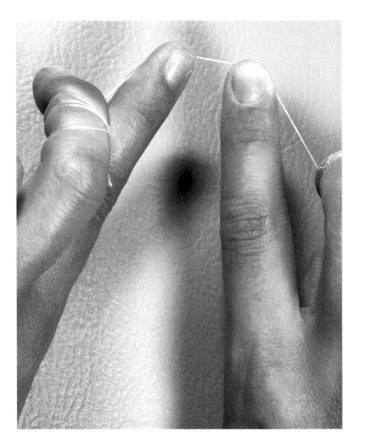

To facilitate its insertion into the spaces between the maxillary or mandibular posterior teeth, the floss is kept between the two extended index fingers.

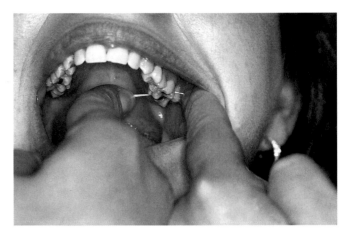

As cleaning is performed, the floss is unwound from the middle finger to the other finger to constantly supply clean floss for each interdental space.

Floss can also be utilized in the form of a loop tied with a knot. In this case, it is no longer necessary to wind the floss around the middle fingers. The fingers of both hands are placed inside the loop and, while the floss is kept taught, a short segment is inserted into the interdental spaces.

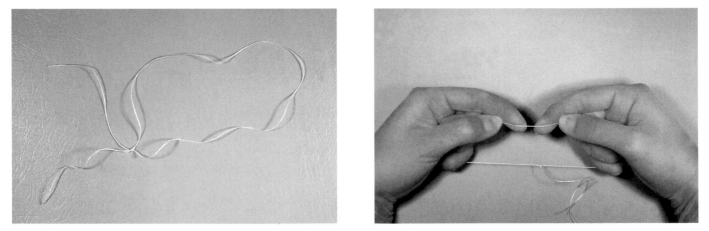

The loop of floss is then rotated to supply a clean segment for each interdental space. This method avoids the gradual tightening of the floss that is wound around the middle fingers and that sometimes causes the patient discomfort.

Floss can also be mounted on a floss holder with an interchangeable spool inserted inside its handle (eg, Glide) to permit the floss to slide so that the segment is always clean and taut. This device facilitates the movement of the floss in the posterior areas because the holder takes the place of the fingers.

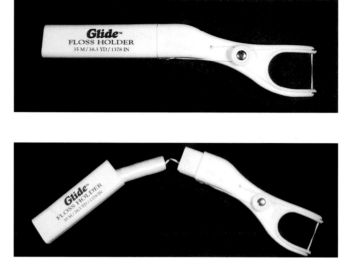

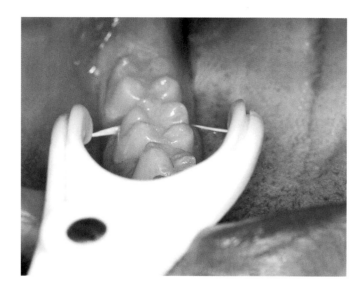

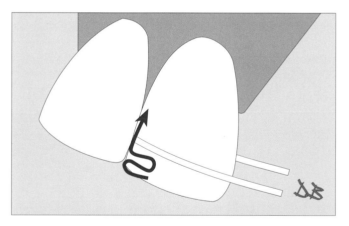

In order to avoid damage to the papillae, the floss is inserted, through the interdental contact point, into the interdental space with a delicate buccolingual movement. Once it has been inserted, it is slid to the gingival margin near the papilla and pulled against the tooth surface in the form of a C.

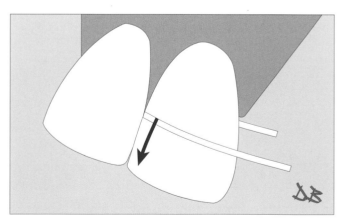

Subsequently, with a vertical movement, the floss is slid from the margin of the papilla to the interdental contact point, repeating this movement several times until the tooth is clean. The surface of the adjacent tooth is cleaned in the same manner, without removing the floss from the interdental space through the contact point.

After cleaning two or three interproximal spaces, the floss is wound to obtain a clean segment for use in the next area.

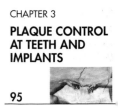
Dental floss is useful in two cases:

1. In narrow spaces between natural teeth

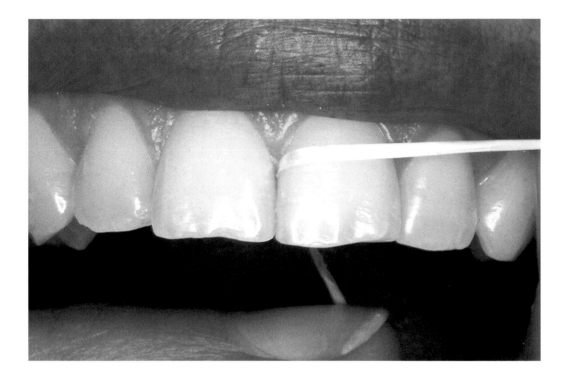

2. In cases in which single implants have been placed

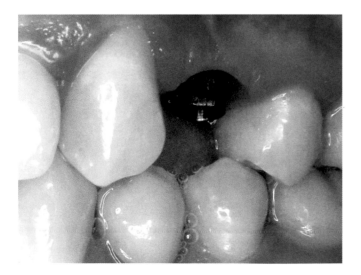 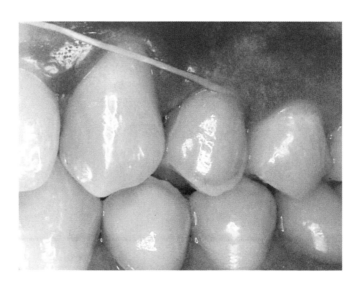

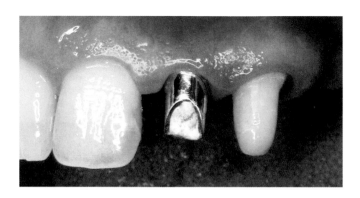

The same procedure is required and effective for the cleaning of interdental spaces both in the presence of prosthetic elements on natural teeth and at implants.

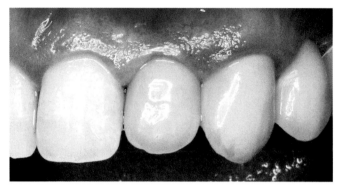

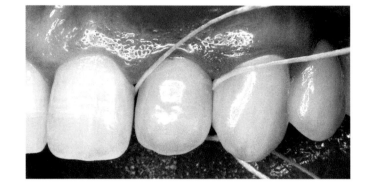

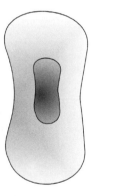

The proper use of dental floss makes it possible to clean almost all interproximal surfaces.[28] It is, however, necessary to bear in mind that dental floss is not effective near concave surfaces (eg, mesial and distal surfaces of roots), for which another type of instrument is more suitable.

Dental floss may damage tissues if it is not used correctly.[12] It is therefore important to review the proper technique for flossing with the patient to arrest the progression of the gingival lesion as soon as it becomes evident that there is tissue damage.

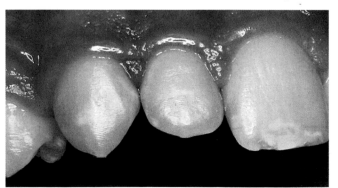

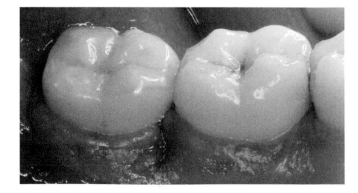

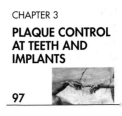
▷ **WOODEN TOOTHPICKS**

Wooden toothpicks may be an excellent substitute for dental floss when the interdental papillae are receded.[21,29] This instrument has a triangular section that is more suitable for interdental spaces, and it is made of soft wood such as birch, lime wood, or balsa (eg, Sanodent, Oral-B; Fresh-Sticks, Paro).

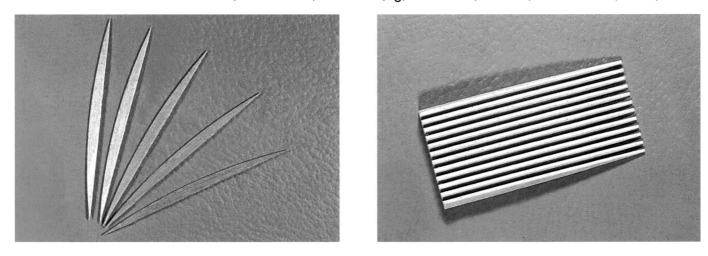

Initially, the toothpick is dampened in the mouth in order to soften it. Then, it is inserted into the interdental space with the base of the triangle turned toward the gingiva. Plaque removal is performed by back-and-forth horizontal movements in the buccolingual direction.

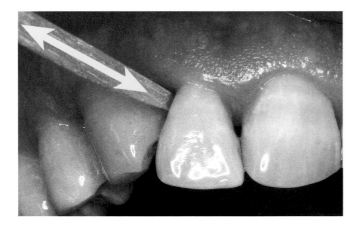

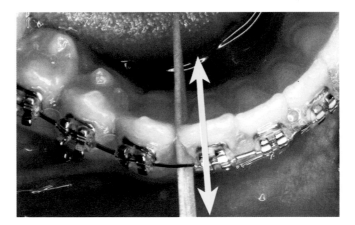

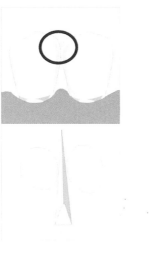

It is, however, necessary to bear in mind that the interdental contact point cannot be cleaned with a toothpick. Furthermore, this instrument must not be used when the papilla is integral because it could cause gingival recession and the formation of a black triangle, which is particularly unesthetic in the anterior regions.

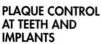
▷ **INTERDENTAL BRUSHES**

Interdental brushes (proxa brushes) are the best choice for cleaning wide interdental spaces. Proxa brushes are available in various forms and dimensions, and the size selected should fill the interdental space as much as possible.[21,29] The proxa brush may be short and inserted into a handle (eg, Butler, Oral-B),

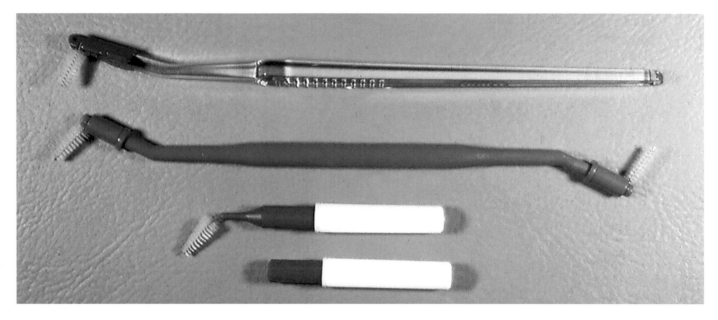

or longer, with a long metal shank that can either act as a handle or be inserted into a special handle (eg, Plak-kontrol, Doft AB, Sweden).

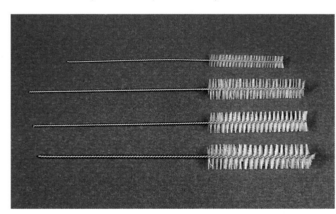

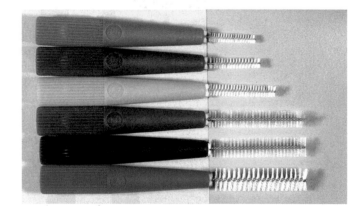

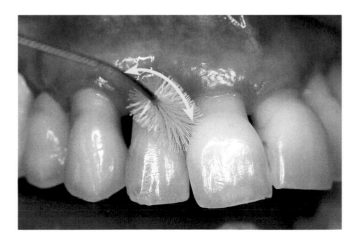

The proxa brush is used according to the same technique utilized with the toothpick: cleaning is accomplished by a back-and-forth movement in the buccolingual direction. Toothpaste is not usually used, but it may be useful for the delivery of antiseptic agents or fluoride in the interdental spaces.

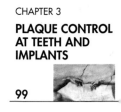
The interdental brush is the ideal instrument for adequate plaque removal in the following cases:

1. In areas in which the root surfaces have a concave outline

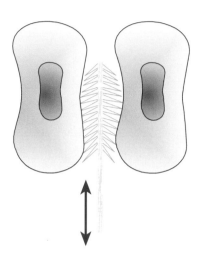

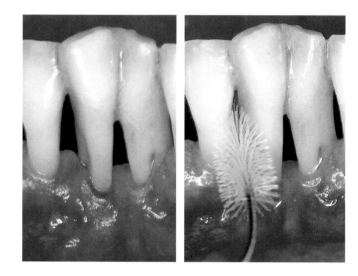

2. In the presence of teeth that have undergone root resection

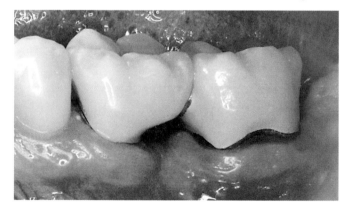

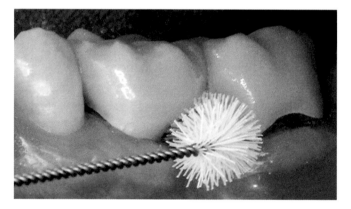

3. In tunnels

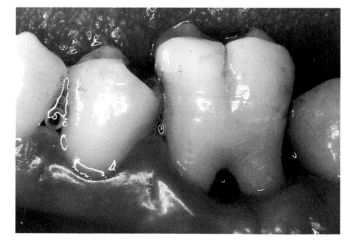

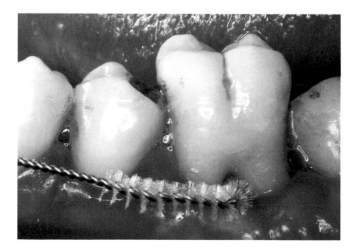

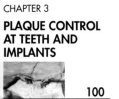
4. In prostheses on natural teeth

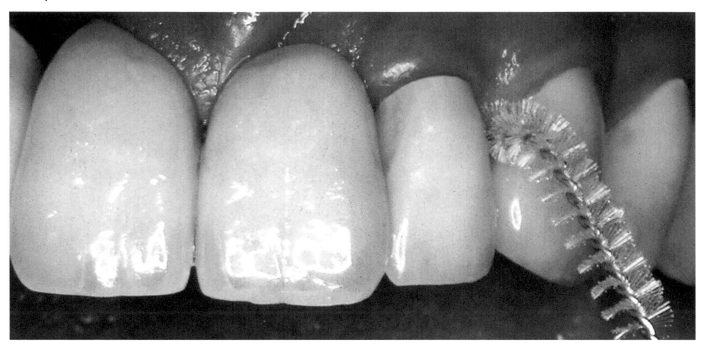

They are also useful in the presence of:

1. Partial or complete-arch prostheses on implants, inserting the proxa brushes both in the buccal and in the lingual directions

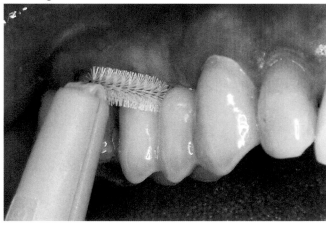

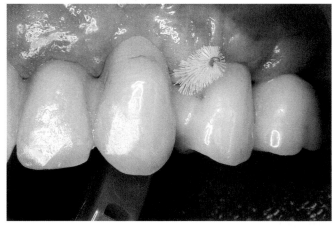

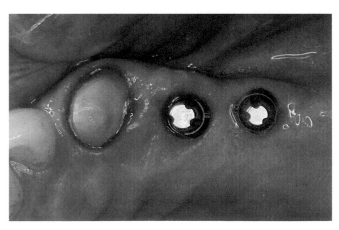

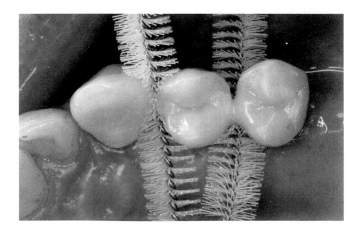

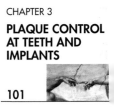
2. Toronto prostheses on implants

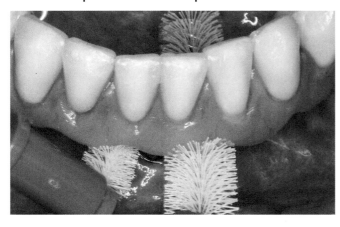

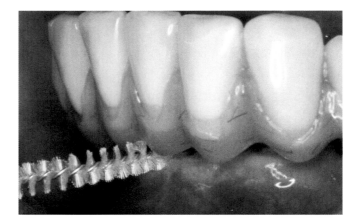

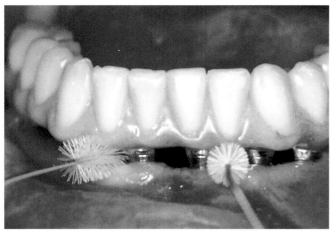

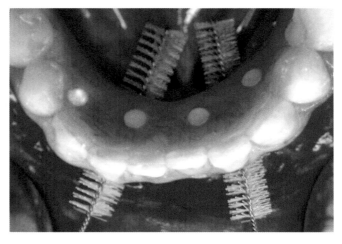

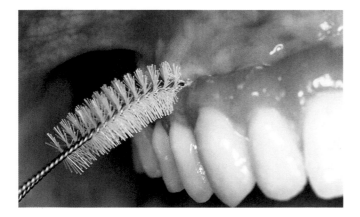

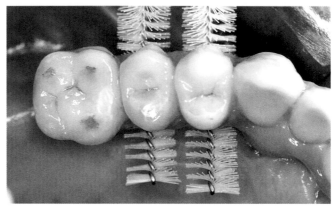

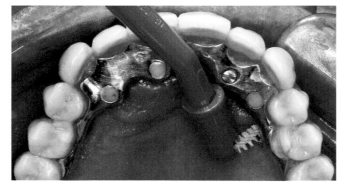

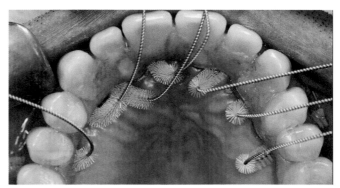

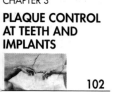
3. Double structures on implants, which are preferred by the prosthodontist when it is necessary to design prosthetic devices that are very high on the buccal side to compensate for loss of hard and soft tissue, and to resolve esthetic and phonetic problems

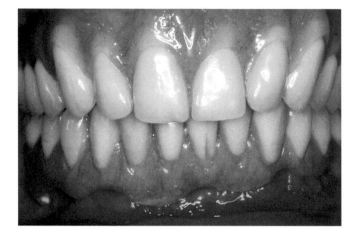

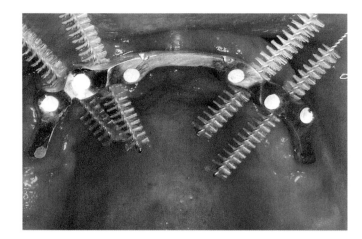

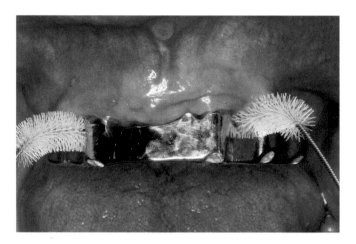

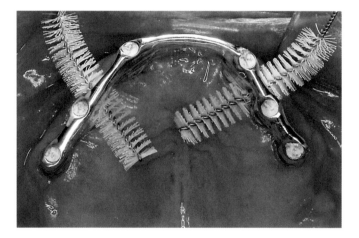

4. Overdentures on natural teeth or implants

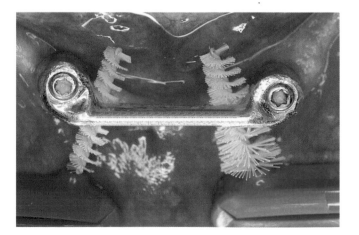

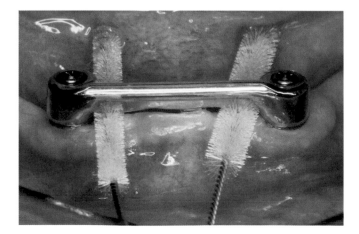

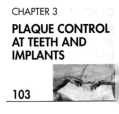
▶ SPECIAL CLEANING DEVICES

Two things are usually sufficient for plaque control: a toothbrush and an interdental instrument. However, in certain situations, other devices and products such as Super-floss (Oral-B), the threader, the single-tufted toothbrush, the perio-aid, the irrigator, the single-tufted electric toothbrush, and mouthrinses may also be necessary and useful.[29]

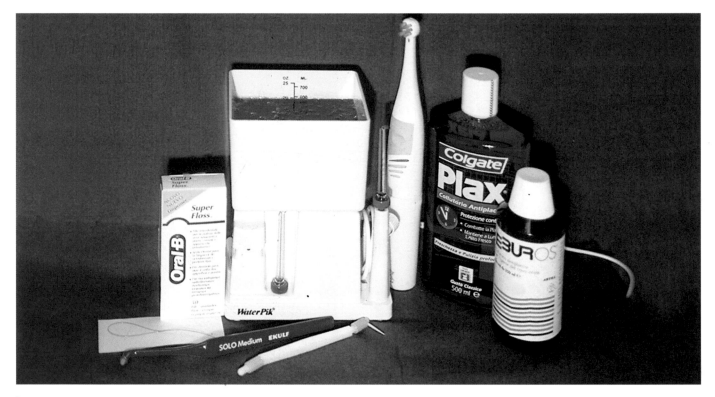

▷ SUPER-FLOSS

Super-floss is a particular type of dental floss that is useful for those who have a prosthesis in which it is necessary to clean the pontics, but in which the insertion of floss through the interdental contact point is not possible.

Super-floss is made up of three sections: a rigid part that serves to insert the floss directly under the prosthesis, a spongy part that serves to clean under the pontics of the bridge, and a part composed of normal floss that is used in the traditional manner.

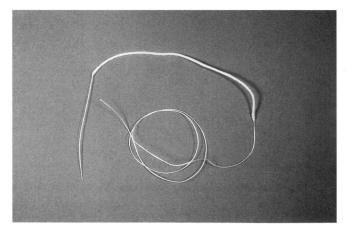

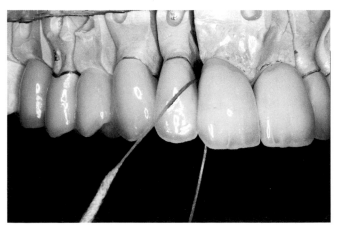

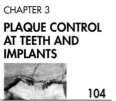
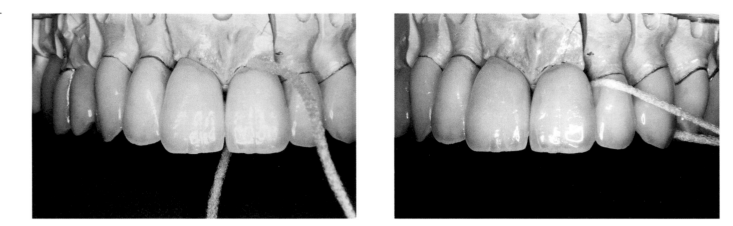

Super-floss may also be useful for patients with complete-arch or Toronto prostheses on implants.

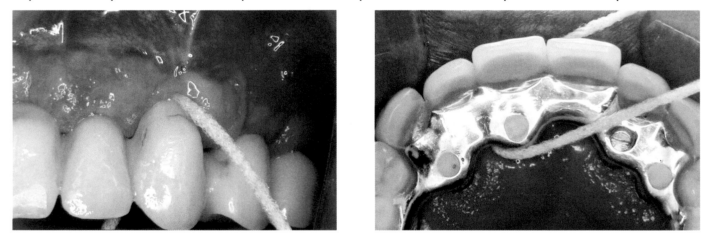

▷ THREADER

A threader is a rigid plastic needle with a very big eye. It is useful for inserting Super-floss under prostheses when the latter present spaces that are too narrow to permit the passage of the rigid part.

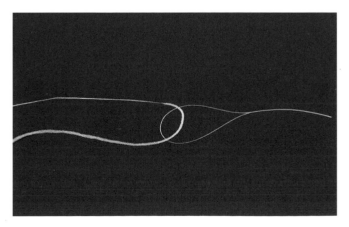
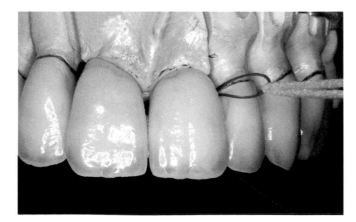

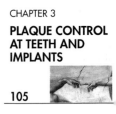

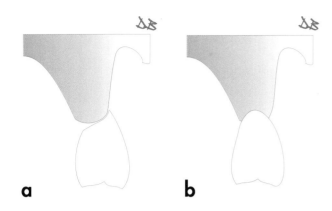

The pontic that is designed to permit the passage of Super-floss usually has a ridge-lap form *(a)*. When, for esthetic reasons, the prosthodontist designs a prosthetic device on natural teeth or implants with ovate pontics *(b)*, it is not necessary for the Super-floss to pass under the pontic.

a   **b**

The patient will use only the instrument that is appropriate to clean the interdental spaces.

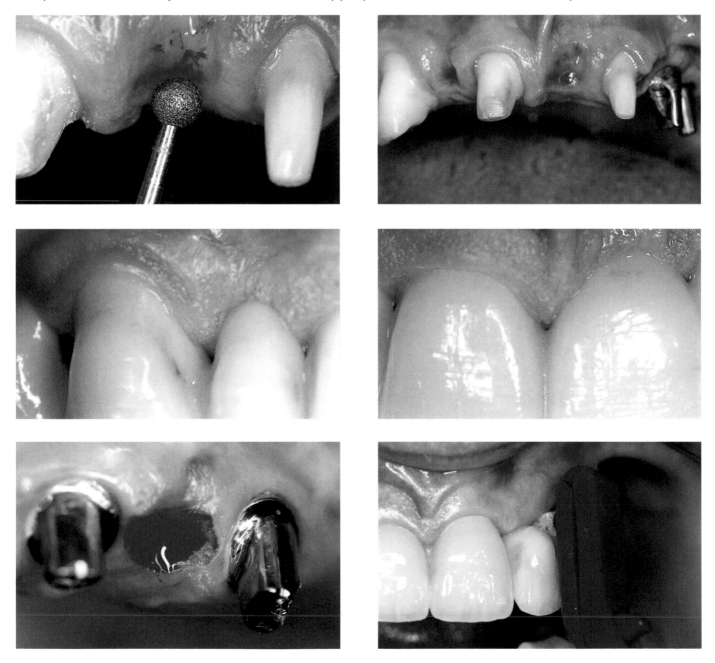

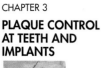
▷ **SINGLE-TUFTED TOOTHBRUSH**

The single-tufted toothbrush has only one tuft of bristles (eg, Tandex SOLO, Ekulf, Sweden) and an angled handle.

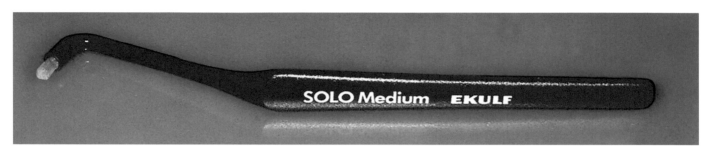

This instrument is inclined at a 45-degree angle toward the gingival sulcus. Then, the Bass technique is performed, using a circular-vibratory movement that is limited to the site in which the brush has been positioned. This adjunctive device is recommended for those areas of the mouth that cannot be easily reached with other hygiene instruments.[21, 29]

It is very useful for cleaning the following areas:

1. The distal surfaces of the last molars

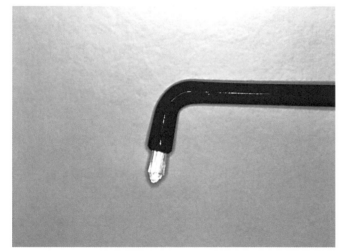

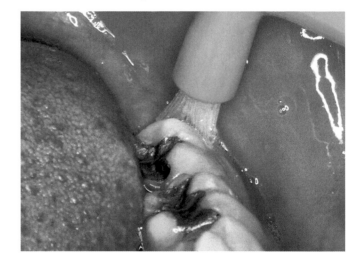

2. Lingual surfaces

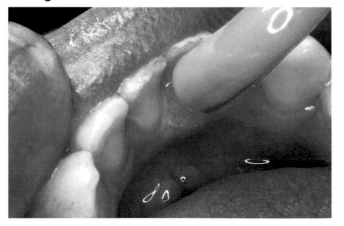

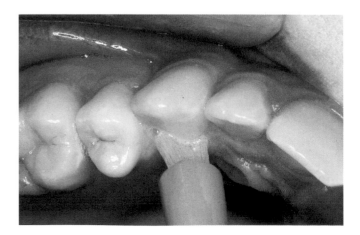

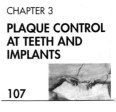
3. Gingival recessions

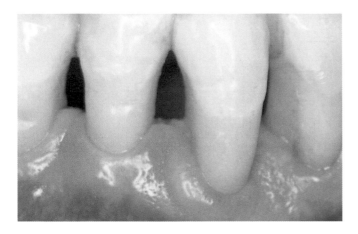 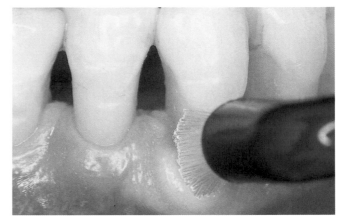

4. Fixed orthodontic appliances

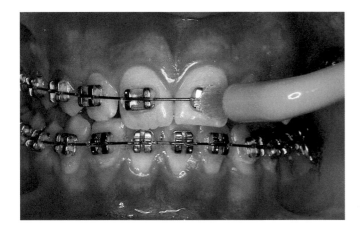 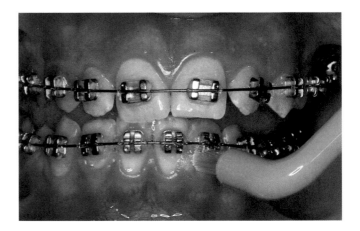

5. Implants

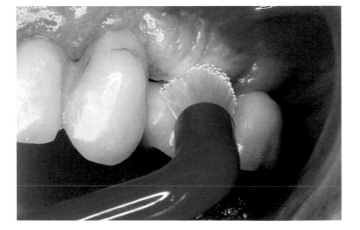 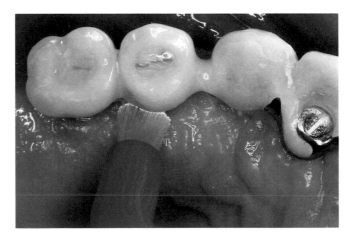

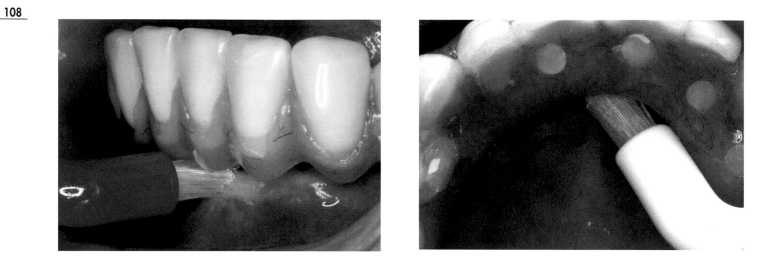

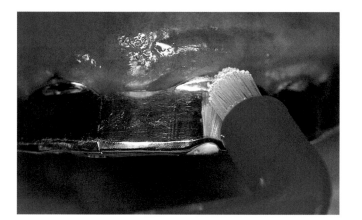

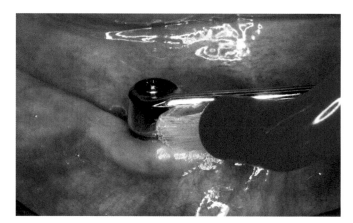

6. The cover screws of implants

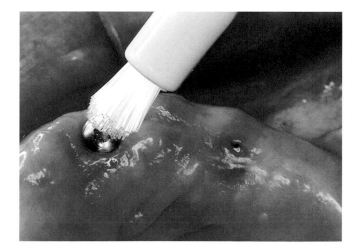

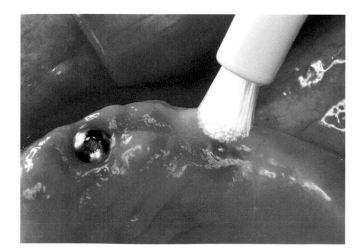

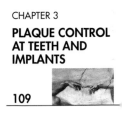
▷ **PERIO-AID**

Perio-aid is a round toothpick inserted in a holder.

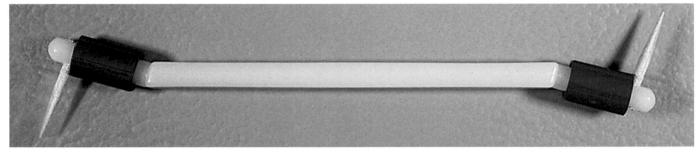

The point of the toothpick is wetted with saliva. Then it is inclined at a 45-degree angle and used with a circular-vibratory movement to remove plaque and clean the area concerned.

The perio-aid can be useful in cleaning recessions, especially clefts, and in situations in which no other instrument, not even the single-tufted brush, fits into the gingival sulcus.

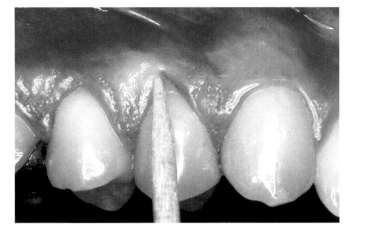 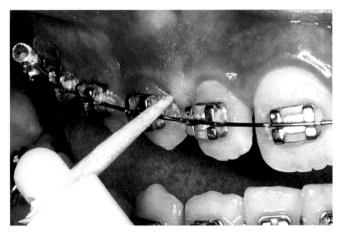

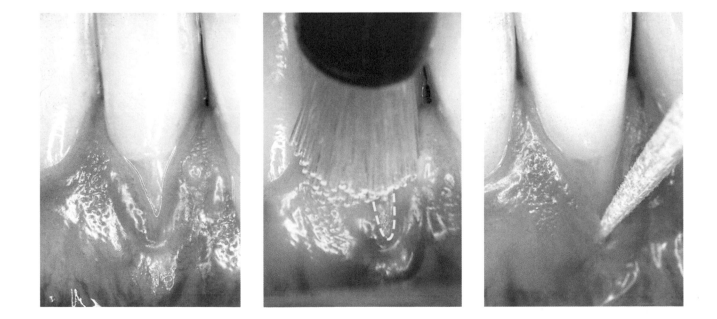

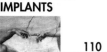
▷ **IRRIGATOR**

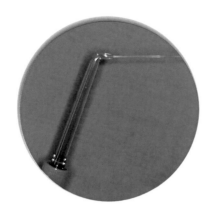

The irrigator (eg, Waterpik oral irrigator, Waterpik Technologies, Fort Collins, CO) is an oral water jet that is effective in removing food debris but is not equally effective on plaque.[29] Consequently, it is not a substitute for the toothbrush or interdental instruments. In fact, findings have revealed that no significant reduction of the Plaque or Gingivitis Index was evidenced in patients who used only these irrigators.[15,27] They can, however, be very useful for patients who have a fixed prosthesis or a fixed orthodontic appliance that renders the removal of debris very difficult.

▷ **SINGLE-TUFTED ELECTRIC TOOTHBRUSH**

The single-tufted electric toothbrush (eg, Rota-dent, Pro-Dentec; Interplak, Conair, East Windsor, NJ) may be a valuable alternative to the manual toothbrush.[29] It is particularly suitable for patients with little manual dexterity, those who are particularly lazy, patients with disabilities, and those with a fixed orthodontic appliance, for whom it is an indispensable aid.[25]

These electric toothbrushes execute a movement that is sufficiently reduced so the brushing they effect is the same as that of the Bass technique performed with a manual toothbrush. Glavind and Zeuner[13] and Baab and Johnson[2] assessed, respectively, the efficacy of the Rota-dent and the Interplak, concluding that the potential of these single-tufted electric toothbrushes to reduce plaque on the tooth surfaces is equal to that of a complete hygiene kit.

The Rota-dent has a single head that rotates, and its structure and function are similar to those of rotating instruments designed for professional use. It is equipped with three types of brushes in different shapes to facilitate access to all areas of the oral cavity.

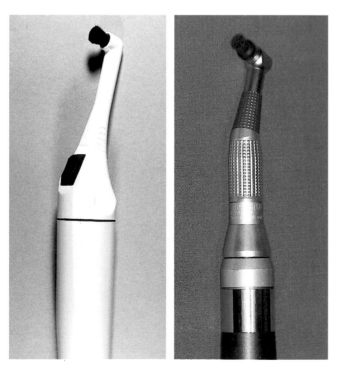

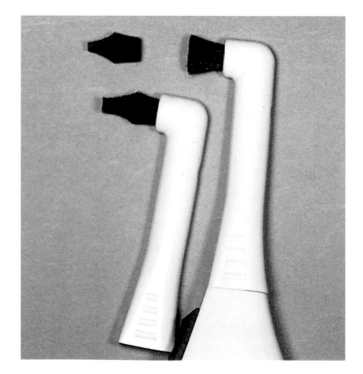

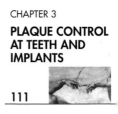
The Interplak electric toothbrush has instead six independent tufts of bristles that perform rotary and counter-rotary movements.

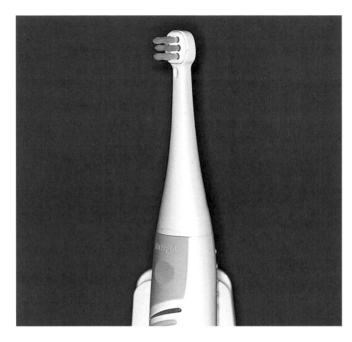

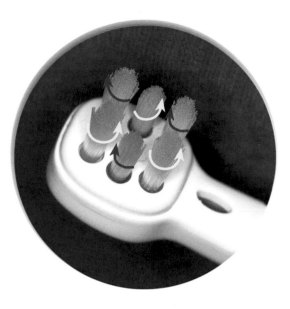

It is useful on natural teeth, in the presence of fixed orthodontic appliances,

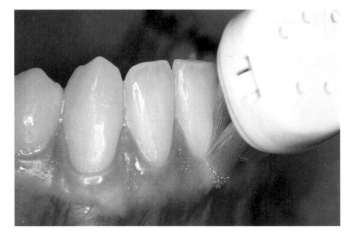

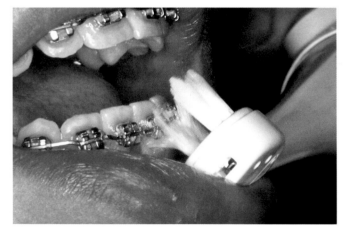

and on prostheses on natural teeth or implants.

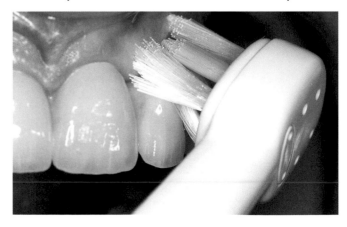

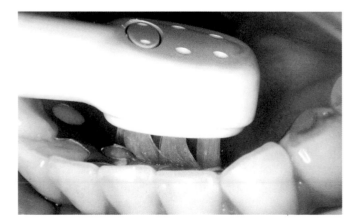

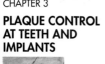
▷ MOUTHRINSES

Mouthrinses can contain different substances that are useful for plaque control in cases in which mechanical cleaning is not possible or is difficult and/or inadequate. Those containing triclosan and the PVM (polyvinyl methyl ether) copolymer, which prolongs the time of retention of triclosan (Plax, Colgate-Palmolive), have given evidence of producing further benefits in oral hygiene and in gingival health if used with normal dental cleaning.[33]

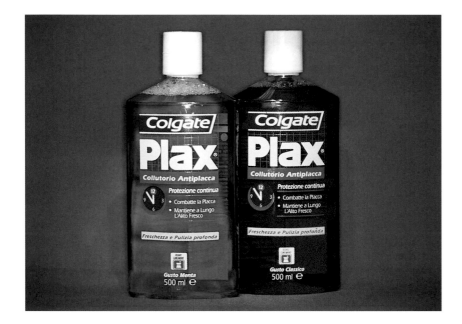

Those containing chlorhexidine (eg, Dentosan and Eburos, Betafarma; Corsodyl, SmithKline Beecham, Philadelphia, PA; Plak-out, Byk Gulden) are excellent for plaque inhibition,[24] but the local side effects, such as pigmentation, limit the prolonged use of this kind of mouthrinse.

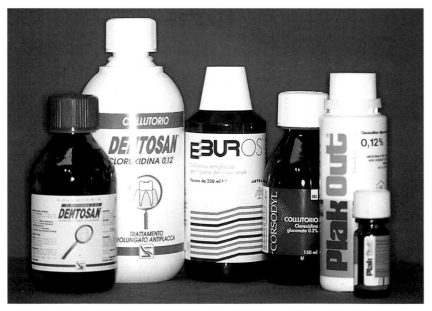

Furthermore, it is necessary to remember that the detergent sodium lauryl sulphate, which is the basic ingredient of toothpastes, reduces the potential of chlorhexidine to inhibit plaque. Therefore, if toothpaste containing sodium lauryl sulphate is used before or after rinsing with this antiseptic, the latter loses its efficacy.[5]

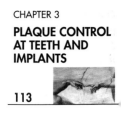
▶ **TABLE OF REFERENCE**

The following table facilitates an appropriate choice of brushing techniques and oral hygiene instruments to be used for plaque removal at teeth and implants in relation to the existing gingival, dental, and prosthetic characteristics.

CLINICAL SITUATION	TECHNIQUES AND INSTRUMENTS
THICK PERIODONTIUM HEALTHY, WITH GINGIVITIS, or WITH PERIODONTITIS	• Short-headed toothbrush • Bass Technique for buccal and lingual surfaces • Horizontal brushing for occlusal surfaces • Interdental instrument: floss, interdental toothpick, or proxabrush chosen in relation to the width of the interdental spaces • Single-tufted toothbrush used with Bass technique, for difficult-to-reach areas, eg, molars and lingual surfaces
THIN PERIODONTIUM HEALTHY or WITH RECESSIONS	• Short-headed toothbrush • Vertical rotary technique for buccal and lingual surfaces • Horizontal brushing for occlusal surfaces • Interdental instrument: dental floss, interdental toothpick, or proxa brush chosen in relation to the width of the interdental spaces • Single-tufted toothbrush used with Bass technique for difficult-to-reach areas, eg, molars and lingual surfaces, and areas in which there are recessions • Perio-aid for clefts

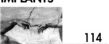
FIXED ORTHODONTIC APPLIANCES

- Single-tufted electric toothbrush or a toothbrush with two rows of tufts
- Bass technique for buccal and lingual surfaces
- Horizontal brushing for occlusal surfaces
- Perio-aid for gingival margin
- Interdental instrument: interdental toothpick or proxa brush chosen in relation to the width of the interdental spaces
- Single-tufted toothbrush used with Bass technique for difficult-to-reach areas, eg, molars and lingual surfaces, gingival margins, and brackets

PROSTHESIS ON NATURAL TEETH

PARTIAL AND COMPLETE-ARCH PROSTHESES

- Short-headed toothbrush
- Bass technique for buccal and lingual surfaces if the periodontium is thick
- Vertical rotary technique for buccal and lingual surfaces if the periodontium is thin
- Horizontal brushing for occlusal surfaces
- Proxa brush
- Super-floss when cleaning of pontics is required
- Threader with Super-floss if the spaces are narrow

PROSTHESIS ON IMPLANTS

SINGLE OR COMPLETE-ARCH PROSTHESES

- Short-headed toothbrush
- Bass technique for buccal and lingual surfaces
- Single-tufted toothbrush with Bass technique for difficult-to-reach areas, eg, molars and lingual surfaces
- Horizontal brushing for the occlusal surfaces of the prosthesis
- Interdental instrument: floss or proxa brush chosen in relation to the width of the interdental spaces
- Super-floss when cleaning of the pontics is required
- Threader with Super-floss if the spaces are narrow

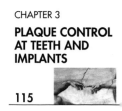
TORONTO PROSTHESES

- Short-headed toothbrush
- Vertical rotary technique for the buccal and lingual surfaces of the prosthesis
- Horizontal brushing for the occlusal surfaces of the prosthesis
- Toothbrush with two rows of tufts or single-tufted toothbrush, with Bass technique, in areas in which there are implants at the level of the peri-implant mucosa
- Proxa brushes of various sizes chosen in relation to the spaces between the abutments and between the peri-implant mucosa and the prosthesis
- Super-floss to clean between the abutments of the prosthesis

DOUBLE STRUCTURES ON IMPLANTS

- Single-tufted toothbrush used with Bass technique along the bar
- Proxa brushes of various sizes chosen in relation to the spaces between the abutments and between the peri-implant mucosa and the bar

OVERDENTURES

- Single-tufted toothbrush around the attachment devices
- Proxa brushes under the bar and near the attachment devices

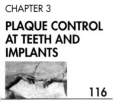
▶ REFERENCES

1. Alexander JF, Saffir AJ, Gold W. The measurement of the effect of toothbrushes on soft tissue abrasion. J Dent Res 1977;56:722–727.

2. Baab DA, Johnson RH. The effect of a new electric toothbrush on subgingival plaque and gingivitis. J Periodontol 1989;60:336–341.

3. Barkvoll P, Rölla G. Triclosan protects the skin against dermatitis caused by sodium lauryl sulphate exposure. J Clin Periodontol 1994;21:717–719.

4. Barkvoll P, Rölla G. Triclosan reduces the clinical symptoms of the allergic patch test reaction (APR) elicited with 1% nickel sulphate in sensitized patients. J Clin Periodontol 1995;22:485–487.

5. Barkvoll P, Rölla G, Svendsen A. Interaction between chlorhexidine digluconate and sodium lauryl sulphate in vivo. J Clin Periodontol 1989;16:593–598.

6. Bass CC. An effective method of personal oral hygiene. J La State Med Soc 1954;106:100–112.

7. Bay I, Kardel KM, Skougaard MR. Quantitative evaluation of the plaque removing ability of different types of toothbrushes. J Periodontol 1967;38:526–533.

8. Bergenholtz A, Britton J. Plaque removal by dental floss or toothpicks. An intra-individual comparative study. J Clin Periodontol 1980;7:516–524.

9. Bergenholtz A, Gustafsson LB, Segerlund N, Hagberg C, Östby N. Role of brushing technique and toothbrush design in plaque removal. Scand J Dent Res 1984;92:344–351.

10. Breitenmoser J, Mörmann W, Muhlemann HR. Damaging effects of toothbrush bristle and form on gingiva. J Periodontol 1979;50:212–216.

11. Charters WJ. Proper home care of the mouth. J Periodontol 1948;19:136–139.

12. Gjermo P, Flötra L. The effect of different methods of interdental cleaning. J Periodontal Res 1970;5:230–236.

13. Glavind L., Zeuner E. The effectiveness of a rotary electric toothbrush on oral cleanliness in adults. J Clin Periodontol 1986;13:135–138.

14. Glaze PM, Wade AB. Toothbrush age and wear as it relates to plaque control. J Clin Periodontol 1986;13:52–56.

15. Hugoson A. Effect of the Water Pik device on plaque accumulation and development of gingivitis. J Clin Periodontol 1978;5:95–104.

16. Keller SE, Manson-Hing LR. Clearance studies of proximal tooth surfaces. Part III and IV: In vivo removal of interproximal plaque. Ala J Med Sci 1969;6:399–405.

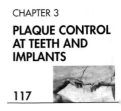

17. Kjaerheim V, Barkvoll P, Waaler SM, Rölla G. Triclosan inhibits histamine-induced inflammation in human skin. J Clin Periodontol 1995;22:423–426.

18. Kreifeldt JG, Hill PH, Calisti LJP. A systematic study of the plaque removal efficiency of worn toothbrushes. J Dent Res 1980;59:2047–2055.

19. Lamberts DM, Wunderlich RC, Caffesse RG. The effect of waxed and unwaxed dental floss on gingival health. Part I. Plaque removal and gingival response. J Periodontol 1982;53:393–399.

20. Lang NP, Cumming BR, Löe H. Toothbrushing frequency as it relates to plaque development and gingival health. J Periodontol 1973;44:396–405.

21. Lindhe J. Clinical Periodontology and Implant Dentistry, ed 3. Copenhagen: Munksgaard, 1997:chap 15.

22. Lindhe J, Rosling B, Socransky SS, Volpe AR. The effect of a triclosan-containing dentifrice on established plaque and gingivitis. J Clin Periodontol 1993;20:327–334.

23. Lobene RR. A clinical study of the anticalculus effect of a dentifrice containing soluble pyrophosphate and sodium fluoride. Clin Prev Dent 1986;8:5–7.

24. Löe H, Schiott CR. The effect of mouthrinses and topical application of chlorhexidine on the development of dental plaque and gingivitis in man. J Periodontal Res 1970;5:79–83.

25. Mantovani S, Clivio A, Fossati C. Indici di placca in pazienti ortodontici: Un nuovo spazzolino elettrico. Dent Cadmos 1996;14:58–64.

26. Massassati A, Frank RM. Scanning electron microscopy of unused and used manual toothbrushes. J Clin Periodontol 1982;9:148–161.

27. Matsuzaki A, Sugano K, Tachibana T, Katano Y, Nahamura J. The effects of toothbrushing and water jetting on oral hygiene. Jpn J Conservative Dent 1974;17:150–153.

28. O'Leary TJ. Oral hygiene agents and procedures. J Periodontol 1970;41:625–629.

29. Rateitschak KH, Rateitschak EM, Wolf HF, Hassel TM. Periodontology, ed 2. Stuttgart: Georg Thieme, 1989:148–157.

30. Sangnes G. Traumatization of teeth and gingiva related to habitual tooth cleaning procedures. J Clin Periodontol 1976;3:94–103.

31. Stilmann PR. A philosophy of the treatment of periodontal disease. Dent Dig 1932;38:314.

32. Waerhaug J. Effect of toothbrushing on subgingival plaque formation. J Periodontol 1981; 52:30–34.

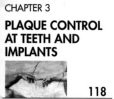
33. Worthington HV, Davies RM, Blinkhorn AS, et al. A six-month clinical study of the effect of a pre-brush rinse on plaque removal and gingivitis. Br Dent J 1993;175:322–329.

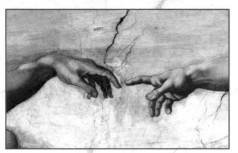

CHAPTER 4

▶ **SCALING AND ROOT PLANING**

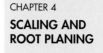
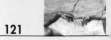
The goal of subgingival surgical instrumentation is to resolve gingival inflammation and to arrest the progressive destruction of the attachment apparatus by removing bacterial plaque and calculus from the gingival pockets; therefore, subgingival debridement and concomitant supragingival plaque control are the most important procedures in the treatment of plaque-associated periodontal disease.[3–7,10,12,16,17,20,21,26,27]

Following are the definitions of a few important terms.

Debridement: Removal of unmineralized bacterial plaque.[15]

Scaling: A procedure that aims to remove calculus (mineralized plaque) from tooth surfaces. Depending on the location of the deposits, scaling may be performed by means of subgingival or supragingival instrumentation.[15]

Root planing: A technique that aims to produce a smooth root surface.

Scaling and root planing may be performed either as nonsurgical or surgical techniques.

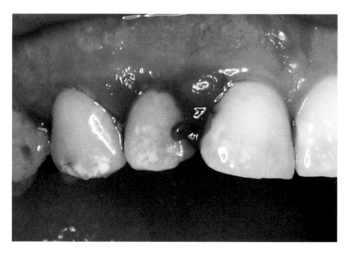

The nonsurgical technique calls for subgingival instrumentation without raising the gingiva. Therefore, it is not possible to have a direct view of the root surface. If the pockets are deep and the treatment plan calls for an attempt to resolve the inflammation with nonsurgical procedures of scaling and root planing, it is necessary to administer local anesthesia in order to perform effective instrumentation without causing the patient pain.

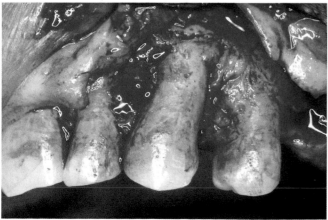

The surgical procedure calls for exposure of the root by means of techniques that make it possible to raise the gingival tissue, thus enabling the operator to obtain a direct view of the root surface and easy access to the area to be treated.

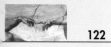
Various types of instruments can be used to perform scaling and root planing effectively.

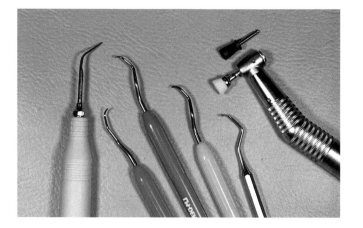

Each operator has a preference, and, after verifying the results obtained with various types of instruments, experience has led me to make choices that I classify and explain as follows:

1. Ultrasonic and sonic instruments

2. Hand instruments

3. Rotating instruments

▶ ULTRASONIC AND SONIC INSTRUMENTS

For many years, ultrasonic instruments have been an effective and rapid aid in cases in which it is necessary to remove gross deposits of calculus that have accumulated over a long period.

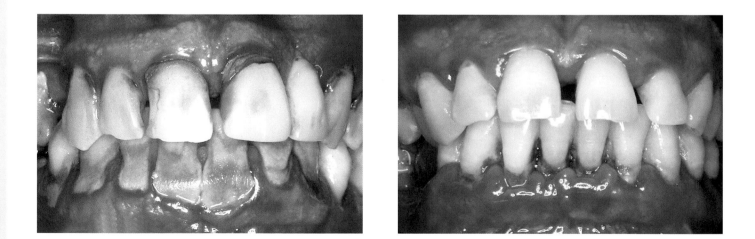

Calculus is usually very thick and tenacious, and its presence may impede adequate periodontal probing. Ultrasonic instruments use high-frequency sound waves that generally range from 25,000 to 45,000 Hz (cycles per second). The vibrations of the tip disintegrate and dislodge the calculus from the tooth surface.

Traditional ultrasonic instruments have very large, bulky points, so their use is limited to the removal of supragingival calculus. It is not possible to use this type of unit to perform adequate subgingival instrumentation.

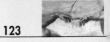
More modern ultrasonic instruments (eg, Amdent 830 or US30, Amdent, Sweden; Slimline, Dentsply, York, PA; Odontoson-M, Goof Denmark, Denmark) have thinner tips that make it easy to reach subgingival areas. I have used the Amdent 830 for a number of years, and I find it a very effective instrument. It works at a frequency that ranges from 24,000 to 28,000 Hz, and tip No. 33 makes it possible to remove calculus in deep pockets.

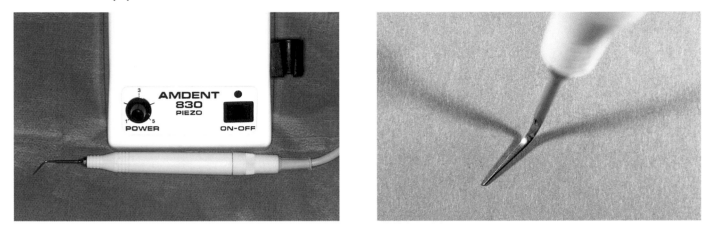

Furthermore, a new instrument for scaling, a "sonic scaler," has recently been introduced (eg, SONICflex 2,000 N, KaVo, Germany). It produces, at the tip, vibrations of sonic frequency that range from 2,300 to 6,300 Hz. Tip No. 8 is designed to facilitate access to subgingival areas.

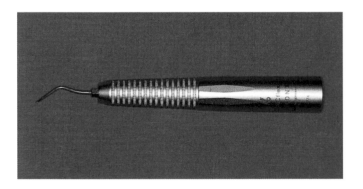

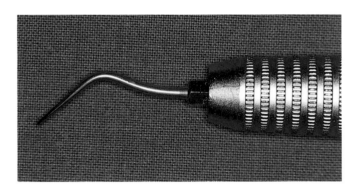

This instrument is particularly suited for the treatment of sites that do not present heavy deposits of calculus, or for treatment during periodic recalls, when there is normally little calculus to remove.

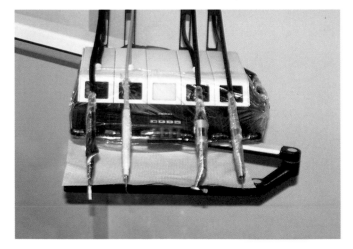

It is advisable to be equipped with both instruments so you can determine which is more suitable for the case under treatment during the appointment. For practical purposes, it is possible to attach both the ultrasonic instrument and the sonic scaler to the dental unit.

Ultrasonic and sonic vibrations produce a considerable amount of heat, so much so that these units are equipped with a water cooling system. Water sprays from a tiny hole near the tip, and at the same time this spray helps to rinse away the deposits that have been dislodged.

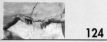
Scaling with ultrasonic instruments often produces an uneven root surface, so it has been suggested that ultrasonic scaling should be supplemented with hand instrumentation to obtain a smoother surface.[8] However, as far as healing is concerned, scaling performed with ultrasonic instruments alone produces the same results as scaling performed with hand instruments.[4,28] Therefore, if properly used, ultrasonic and sonic instruments must be regarded not only as adjuncts, but also as valid substitutes for hand instruments. Furthermore, they may be the best choice for scaling at furcation areas.[14] Since, however, it is not easy to reach all areas of the mouth adequately with ultrasonic and sonic instruments, it is advisable to integrate their use with that of hand instruments.

▷ USE OF ULTRASONIC AND SONIC INSTRUMENTS

Because the deposits of calculus are removed by the vibrations of the tip, the operator who uses this instrument must apply very light pressure, constantly moving the tip in circular strokes while keeping it parallel to the surface in order to prevent damage to the tooth structure.

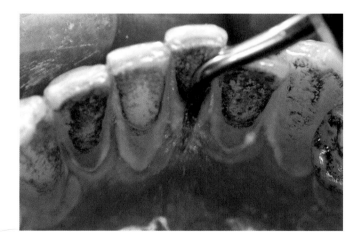 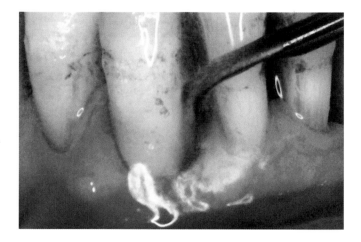

The proper use of ultrasonic instruments enables the operator to remove gross deposits of calculus rapidly.

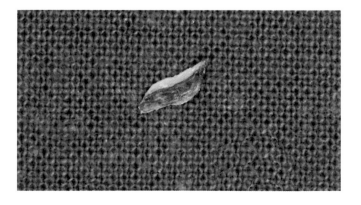 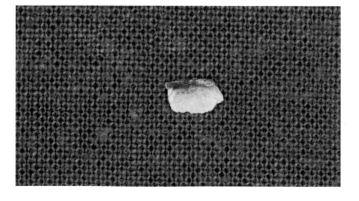

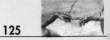
▶ HAND INSTRUMENTS

These instruments are used both for supragingival and subgingival scaling and for root planing. Various types of instruments of different shapes and sizes are available on the market, but, on the basis of personal experience, individual operators should choose a limited series of instruments that can help them to perform their work most effectively. Thorough knowledge of the characteristics of instruments is of essential importance because it will facilitate operators' efforts to learn the proper techniques for their use. Once these techniques have been acquired, operators will use the instruments competently, without lacerating the soft tissue or causing pain if the instrumentation is being performed at a depth that does not require local anesthesia.

▷ GENERAL CHARACTERISTICS OF HAND INSTRUMENTS

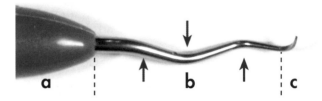

In general, hand instruments are made of stainless steel and are composed of three parts: *(a)* the handle, *(b)* the shank, and *(c)* the working part (blade).[13]

The handle is available in various sizes, shapes, and surfaces. Ribbed or silicone handles enable the operator to maintain a firmer grasp and prevent the instrument from slipping. Fairly large handles provide a more comfortable grasp. The handles may also be color coded to permit rapid and precise identification of each instrument.

The shank is the part of the instrument that unites the working part to the handle. It may have more or less accentuated angulations, designed to permit access to the various dental surfaces. An instrument with a straight shank is usually used on anterior teeth, while an instrument with a very angled shank is used on posterior teeth. The length of the shank may also vary; long shanks are necessary for the treatment of deep periodontal pockets.

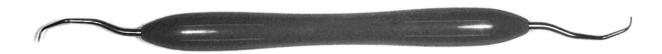

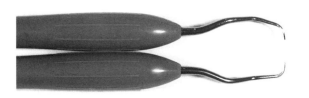

The working part (blade), the final extremity of the instrument, effectively executes the scaling. Generally, instruments have two working parts with mirror-turned blades situated at the opposite ends of the handle. The working part of the curette and the sickle have different features.

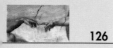
▷ THE UNIVERSAL CURETTE AND THE SICKLE

The working part of the universal curette is semicircular and is composed of [9,13]:

- A facial surface
- Two flat lateral surfaces
- A rounded back
- Two cutting edges that converge to form a rounded toe

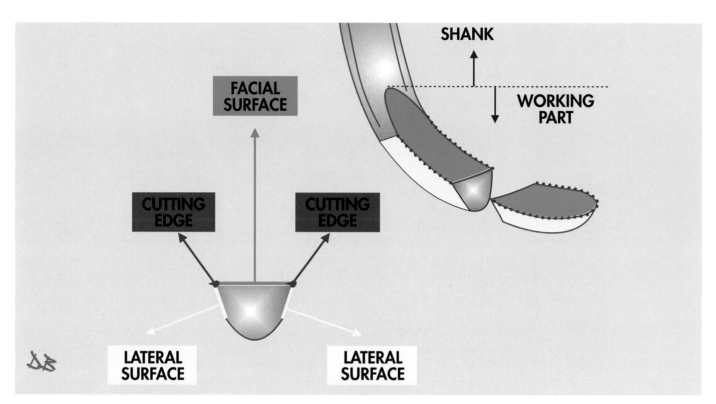

The working part of the sickle has the form of a scythe. It has a triangular cross section and comprises:

- A facial surface
- Two lateral surfaces that are not flat but slightly curved
- A slightly beveled back
- Two cutting edges that converge to form a sharp toe

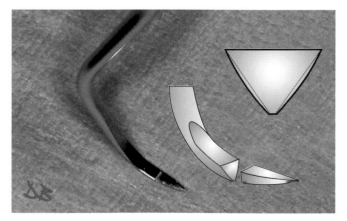

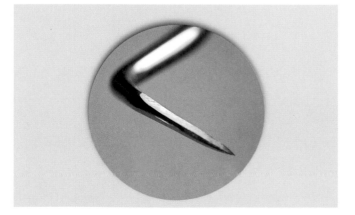

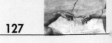
The universal curette (eg, M23A, Deppeler, Switzerland) can be used "universally" on all dental surfaces;

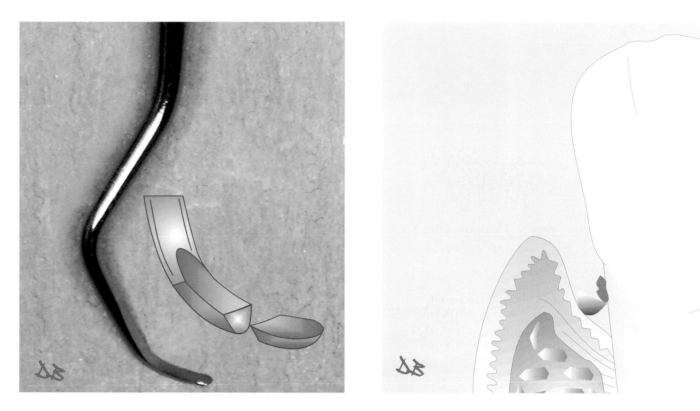

has two parallel cutting edges of equal length that make it possible to work on both mesial and distal surfaces utilizing the same end of the instrument; and has the facial surface of the working part positioned perpendicular (90 degrees) to the final part of the shank.

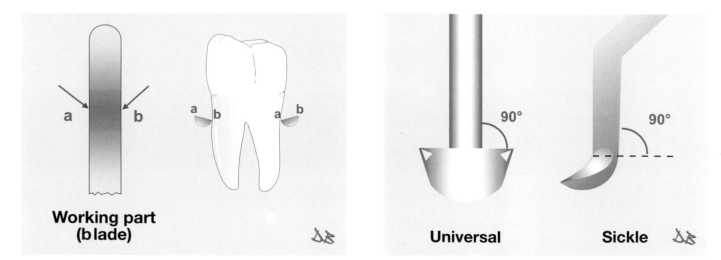

As far as these three aspects are concerned, the universal curette may be considered similar to the sickle (eg, M23, Deppeler; LM23 or Mini Sickle, LM Dental, Finland) because the latter also has two cutting edges and the working part is perpendicular to the final part of the shank. The universal curette and the sickle are easy to use in periodontal treatment of gingivitis and shallow pockets. In these cases, I personally choose the sickle.

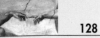
▷ GRACEY CURETTES

Gracey curettes (eg, Gracey, LM Dental) are instruments that are easy to use, and for this reason they are the ones I prefer for periodontal treatment in deep pockets.

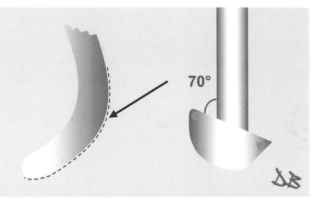

These instruments have a curved working part and only one cutting edge; the facial surface of the working part offset at 70 degrees with respect to the lower part of the shank (this inclination makes it possible to insert the blade easily and rapidly into the gingival pocket in the correct working position with respect to the root); and a specific shank angulation for the various dental surfaces (this enables the operator to reach areas where access is limited).

Generally, Gracey curettes with shanks bent in several severe angles are more suited for posterior teeth. The complete series of Gracey curettes is composed of nine double-ended instruments, two of which were recently added.

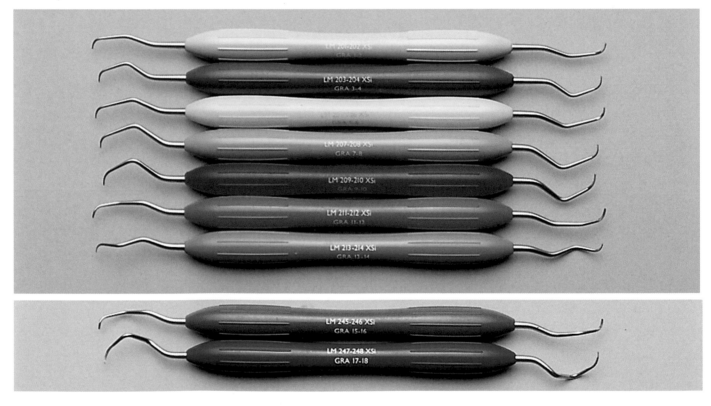

Gracey 1/2: Buccal surfaces of anterior teeth
Gracey 3/4: Lingual surfaces of anterior teeth
Gracey 5/6: Surfaces of premolars
Gracey 7/8: Buccal and lingual surfaces of molars
Gracey 9/10: Buccal and lingual surfaces of molars (shank with more acutely angled bends)
Gracey 11/12: Mesial surfaces of molars
Gracey 13/14: Distal surfaces of molars
Gracey 15/16: Mesial surfaces of molars (shank with more acutely angled bends)
Gracey 17/18: Distal surfaces of molars (shank with more acutely angled bends)

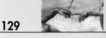
It is not necessary to use all the Gracey curettes; for practical purposes, four curettes from the entire set are sufficient to enable the operator to reach all areas of the oral cavity.[13]

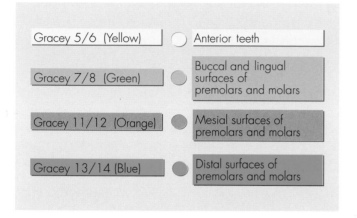

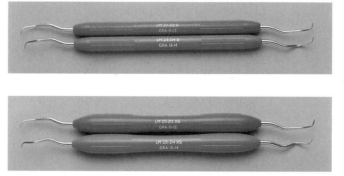

The 11/12 and the 13/14 are the fundamental curettes.

Although Dr Gracey devised these curettes for use in specific areas, it is possible to use them in other areas as well once the general principles for their use have been understood and applied.

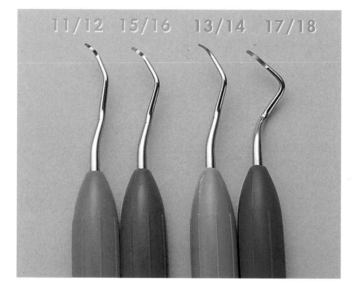

In certain situations, the two newest curettes make work more comfortable for the operator. In fact, the 15/16 and 17/18 present a more accentuated angulation of the shank, making it possible for the operator to instrument the posterior areas more easily, without interfering with the handle in the opposite arch. The design of these two curettes is particularly useful when the patient's mouth cannot be opened sufficiently.

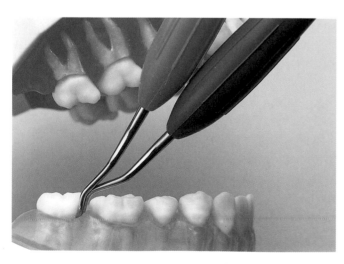

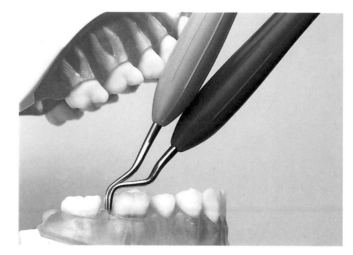

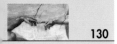
HOW TO IDENTIFY THE CUTTING EDGE OF GRACEY CURETTES

The operator must be able to recognize the cutting edge of the Gracey curette to be able to insert it properly into the periodontal pocket and sharpen it correctly. The most traditional and common method for identifying the cutting edge is to observe the shank of the instrument and to position the lower part of the shank, that is, the segment nearest to the working part, perpendicular to a level surface. The facial surface will not be parallel to the plane surface but oblique; therefore, an upper edge and a lower edge will be easily recognized: the lower edge is always the cutting edge.

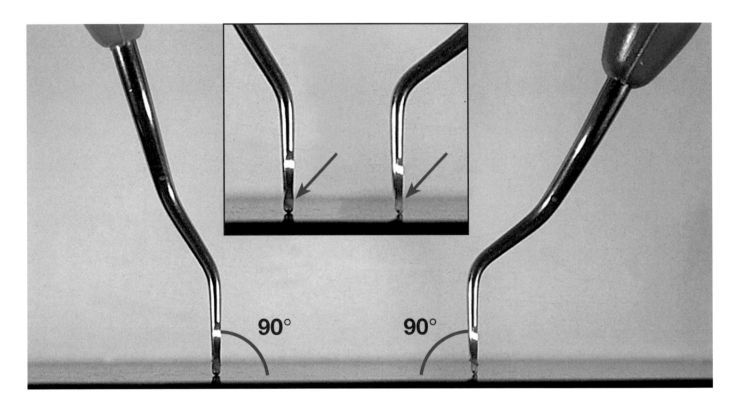

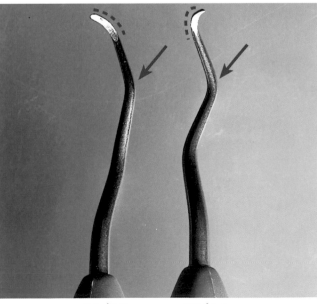

There is an easier and more practical method for recognizing the cutting edge of the 11/12 and the 13/14. The shanks of these two curettes present more bends but, for each extremity, the bend nearest to the working part is one that must be observed.

The cutting edge of the 11/12 is always on the same side as the bend nearest to the working part.

The cutting edge of the 13/14 is always on the side opposite the bend nearest to the working part.

11/12   13/14

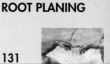
▷ GRASP OF THE INSTRUMENT AND FINGER RESTS

It is necessary to bear in mind that instruments for scaling and root planing must be used with a certain amount of pressure in very narrow spaces without damaging the surrounding tissue. Therefore, indispensable elements for optimum instrumentation are: a correct grasp, a proper and stable finger rest, and effective strokes.

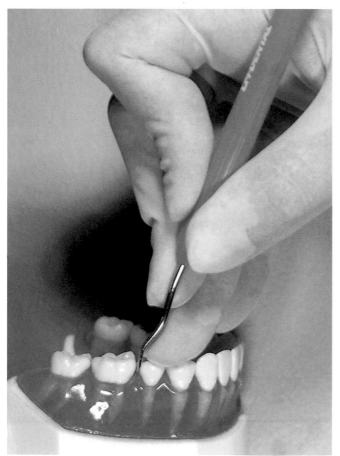

In order to achieve a firm grip and a stable guide, a modified "pen grasp" must be used.[9,13,24]
- The instrument is held between the thumb, the index finger, and the middle finger, which rests on the shank.
- The middle finger is extended, and the fingertip is placed on the side of the first part of the shank near the handle.
- The index finger is bent and slid backward on the handle.
- The thumb is bent and positioned on the opposite side of the handle, midway between the index and the middle fingers.

The "triangular" position of the fingers locks the curette as if it were in a vice, providing a firm guide, better control of the instrument, and a greater tactile sensitivity. The finger rest must be as close as possible to the working area. The ring finger is used for this purpose, and the middle finger may rest against it.

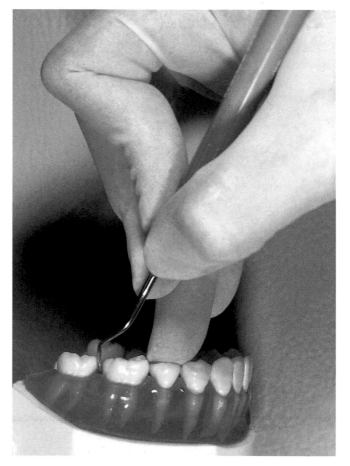

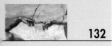
A finger rest must be established in all cases, no matter what area is being treated, what instrument has been chosen, and whether the operator prefers a direct or indirect view of the site to be treated.

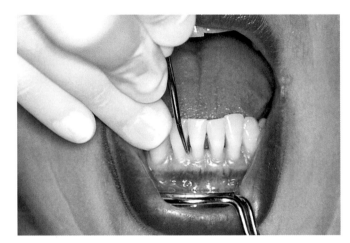 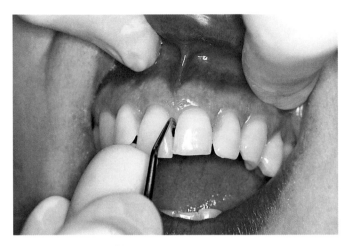

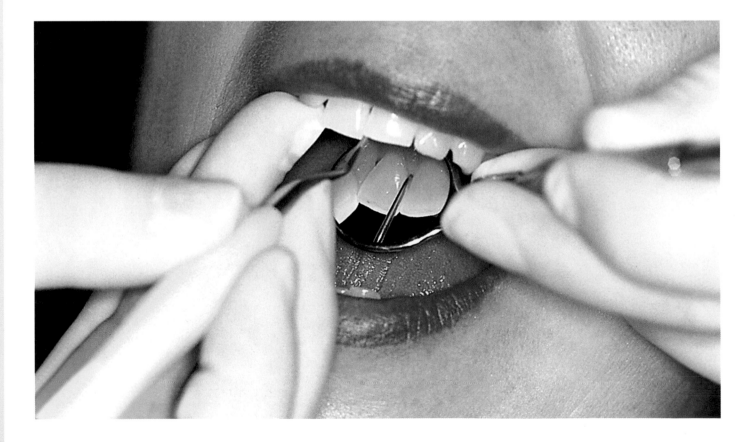

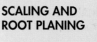
In order to perform more effective instrumentation, in certain situations the operator may be obliged to establish a finger rest that is not exactly close to the working area.

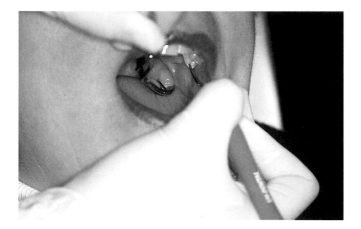

For example, an extraoral rest may be necessary, either on the chin so that the palm of the hand cups the mandible,

or on the reinforcing finger of the nonworking hand that pulls back the cheek and at the same time pushes against the shank of the curette, thus increasing the pressure applied on the tooth surface during instrumentation.

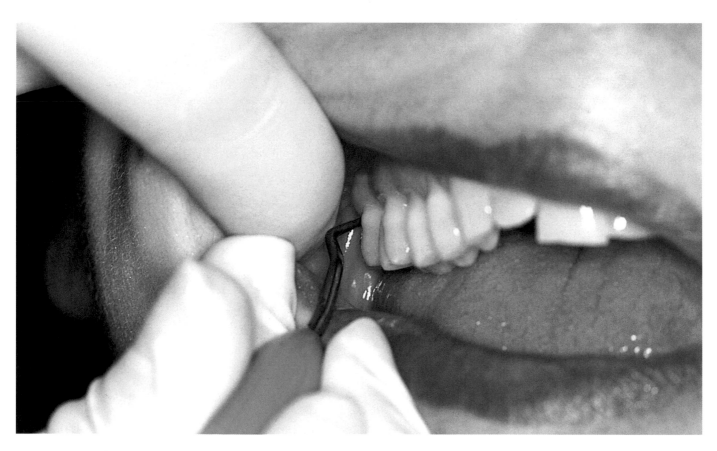

Whichever the choice, the most important thing is to establish and maintain a stable rest to permit a controlled and efficient removal of calculus.

▷ **POSITION OF THE OPERATOR**

The operator must work in different positions in relation to the patient to be able to reach and treat the various areas of the mouth. Operators must choose the positions that they find most comfortable and that enable them to easily reach the areas to be treated and to work in most cases with a direct view. A direct view is useful in treating the lingual surfaces of incisors and the distal surfaces of molars.

The right-handed operator will use positions that are different from those used by an operator who is left-handed or ambidextrous.[9,24,25] Below, I suggest the positions that I consider the most comfortable to reach all areas of the oral cavity. If the suggested positions are utilized, the operator can avoid continuously moving the patient's head while attempting to obtain an adequate view of the area under treatment.

RIGHT-HANDED OPERATORS

In terms of the face of a clock, the positions of the right-handed operator are:

1. At 8 o'clock, in front of the patient

2. At 9 o'clock, beside the patient

3. At 11, 12, or 1 o'clock, behind the patient

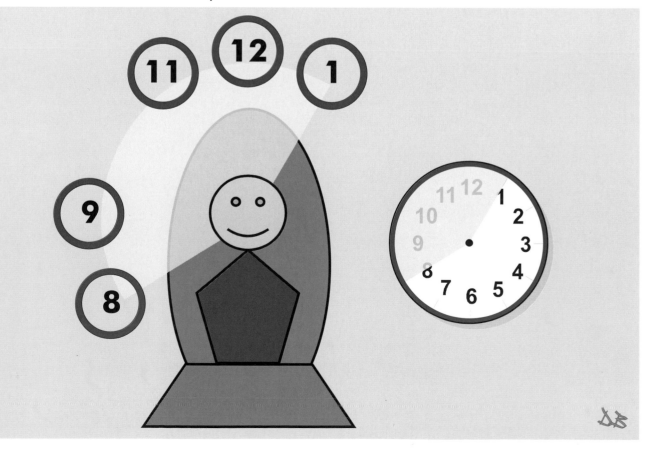

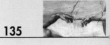
The right-handed operator can treat all surfaces of the incisors of both arches by assuming positions that correspond to 9 and 12 o'clock.

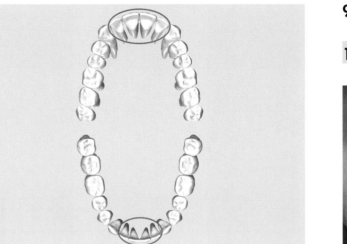

9 o'clock: 12 and 11 distal, 21 and 22 mesial, 42 and 41 distal, 31 and 32 mesial

12 o'clock: 12 and 11 mesial, 21 and 22 distal, 42 and 41 mesial, 31 and 32 distal

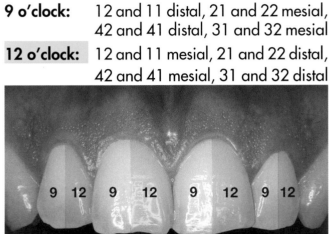

In order to reach posterior teeth from canines to third molars, the right-handed operator may work in different positions according to the surfaces to be treated. The diagrams below indicate the various surfaces to be treated and the positions that are useful for the right-handed operator.

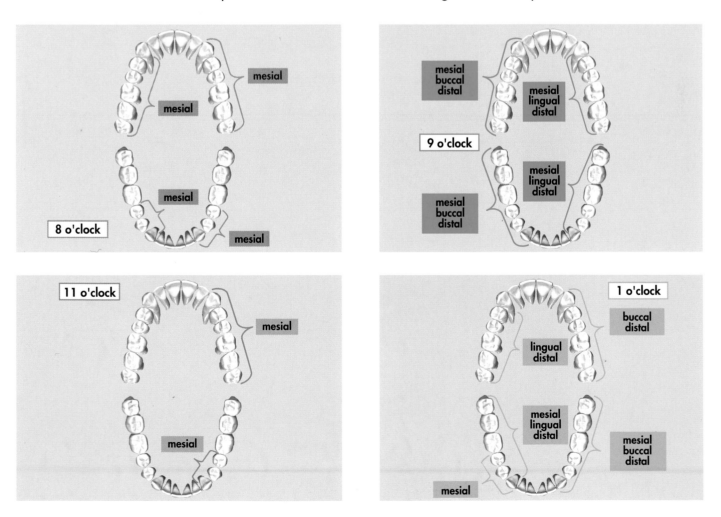

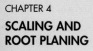
LEFT-HANDED OPERATORS

The left-handed operator works in positions that are the opposite of those used by the right-handed operator:

1. At 4 o'clock, in front of the patient

2. At 3 o'clock, beside the patient

3. At 1, 12, or 11 o'clock, behind the patient

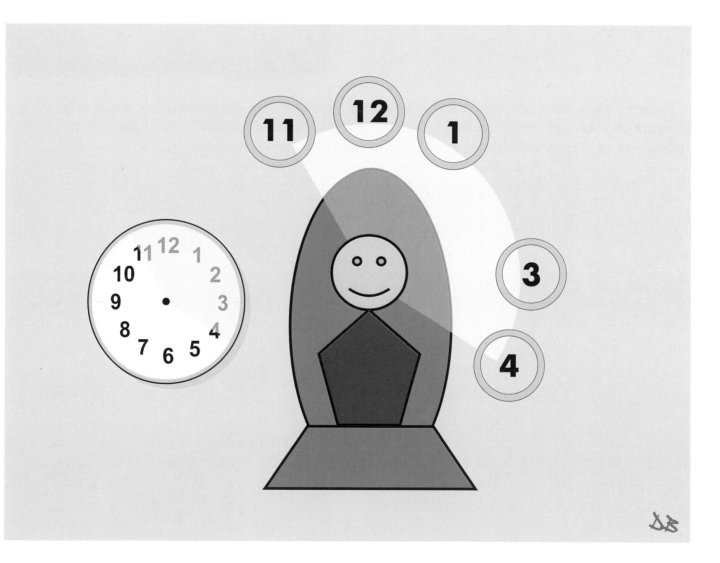

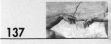
The left-handed operator can treat all surfaces of the incisors of both arches by working in positions that correspond to 3 and 12 o'clock.

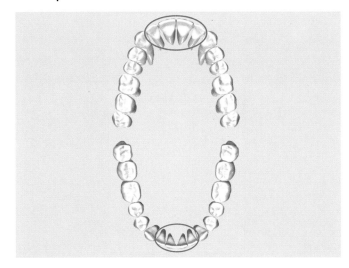

3 o'clock: 22 and 21 distal, 11 and 12 mesial, 32 and 31 distal, 41 and 42 mesial

12 o'clock: 11 and 12 distal, 22 and 21 mesial, 41 and 42 distal, 32 and 31 mesial

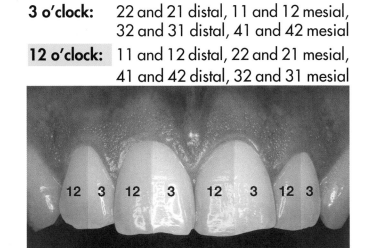

In order to reach the posterior teeth from canines to third molars, the left-handed operator may assume different positions according to the surfaces to be treated. The diagrams below indicate the various surfaces to be treated and the positions that are useful for the left-handed operator.

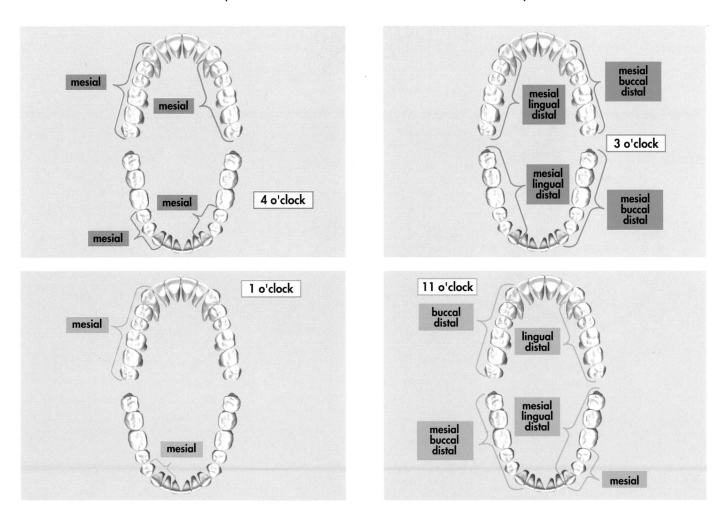

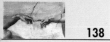

AMBIDEXTROUS OPERATORS

The ambidextrous operator has many advantages, because the ability to alternate the right hand with the left permits them to choose the most comfortable working position for each area to be treated, almost always allowing them to work with a direct view:

1. At 9 o'clock, beside the patient

2. At 12 o'clock, behind the patient

3. At 3 o'clock, beside the patient

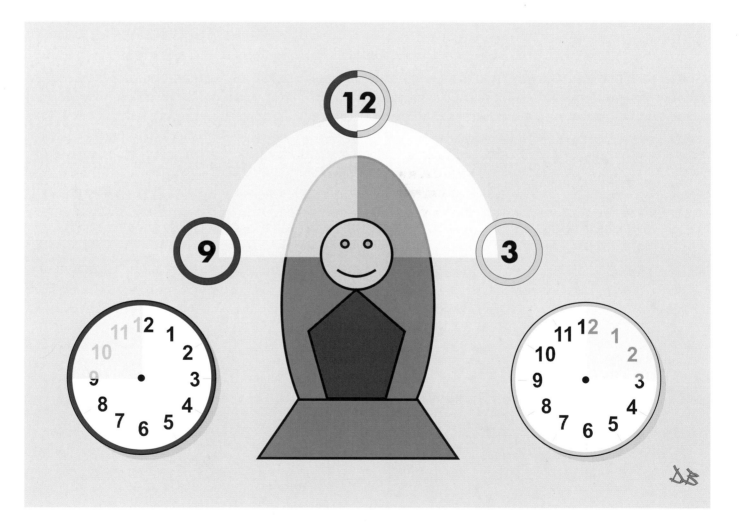

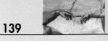
While remaining in the 12 o'clock position, the ambidextrous operator can reach and treat the surfaces of the incisors in both arches by simply changing hands as indicated below:

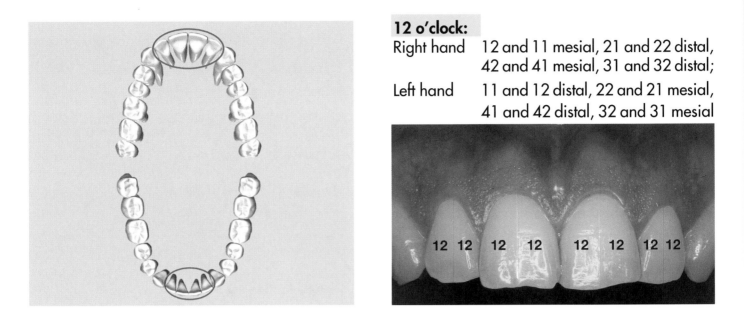

12 o'clock:

Right hand	12 and 11 mesial, 21 and 22 distal, 42 and 41 mesial, 31 and 32 distal;
Left hand	11 and 12 distal, 22 and 21 mesial, 41 and 42 distal, 32 and 31 mesial

In order to reach the posterior teeth from canines to third molars, the ambidextrous operator may assume different positions according to the surfaces to be treated, using one hand or the other. Ambidextrous operators must move from the right to the left of the patient in order to obtain the utmost advantage from their particular ability. The following diagrams indicate the various surfaces to be treated and the positions that are useful for the ambidextrous operator (9 o'clock when the right hand is used and 3 o'clock when the left hand is used). As can be seen, the ambidextrous operator is able to reach all of the posterior dental surfaces from these two positions. Naturally, in certain circumstances, the ambidextrous operator may also find it helpful to use the other positions normally assumed by right-handed and left-handed operators.

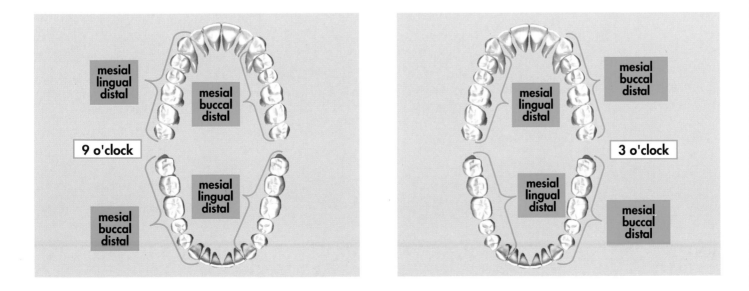

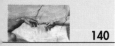
▷ USE OF GRACEY CURETTES

Before using curettes, the probing depth is established with the periodontal probe. In order to perform effective treatment, the operator must have sufficient tactile sensitivity to locate the accumulation of subgingival calculus, "feeling" the vibrations transmitted from the tip to the handle of the probe. This sensation can be perceived only if the grasp is light: a hard, solid resistance indicates the presence of calcifications that must be removed with the appropriate instruments. The suitable sharp curette is chosen, and proper scaling procedures are performed.[9,13,24,25]

The working part of the curette is inserted into the periodontal pocket, maintaining the facial surface of the instrument as parallel as possible to the tooth surface *(A)*. In this way, the last part of the shank will be oblique. This procedure will establish an angulation of approximately 0 degrees with respect to the tooth surface, and the grasp must be light (as when using the periodontal probe). This exploratory stroke performed with the curette is used to reach the bottom of the sulcus or pocket. The operator must then use tactile sensitivity to detect deposits of calculus.

The grasp of the instrument is then tightened, and the working part is "opened" by moving the last part of the shank away from the tooth until the working part is parallel to the root surface and the angle between the facial surface of the blade and the root surface is 70 degrees *(B)*.

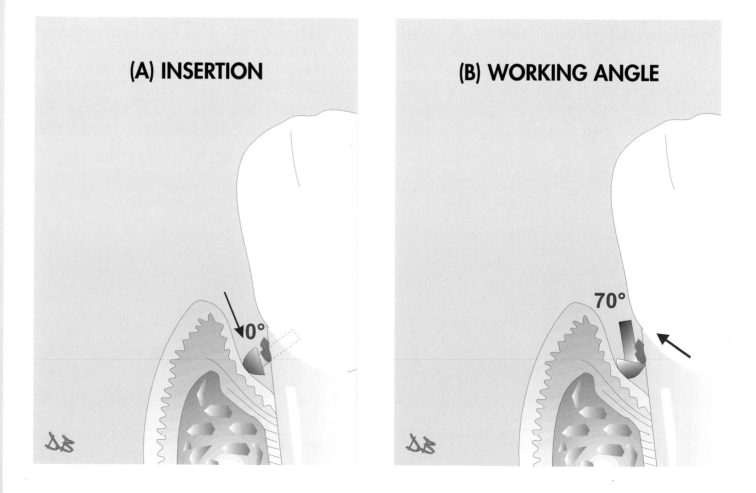

(A) INSERTION

(B) WORKING ANGLE

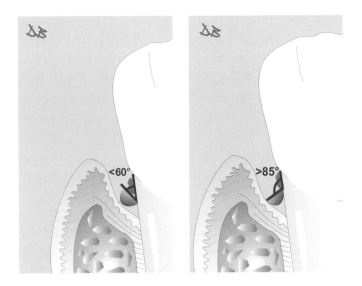

A certain tolerance, which ranges from 60 to 85 degrees, exists.

If the angle were opened to less than 60 degrees, the cutting edge would not effectively remove the deposit but would simply "burnish" it, leaving thin, smooth sheets of calculus that are very difficult to detect with the probe. The presence of this calculus might jeopardize the results of the periodontal treatment.

If the angle were opened to more than 85 degrees, the edge opposite the working part might lacerate and remove some soft tissue despite the fact that it is a safe edge.

Therefore, in order to perform effective instrumentation, it is necessary to position the curette so that the facial surface is at an angle of 70 degrees with respect to the root surface.

Maintaining this working angulation, lateral pressure is applied against the root of the tooth, using almost exclusively the lower third of the working part. If the intermediate part is used, the tip will lacerate the soft tissue.[9]

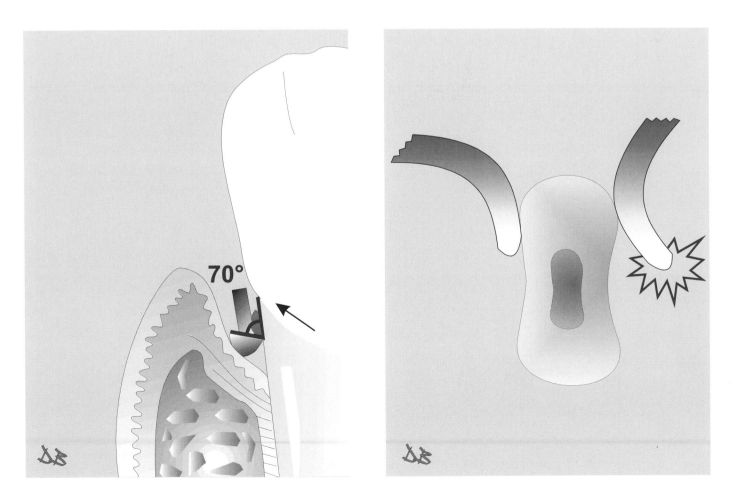

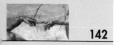
(C) PULL STROKE (SCALING)

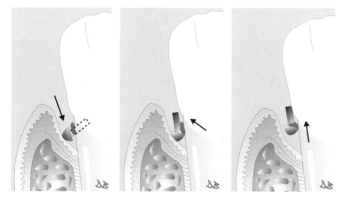

Then, with a firm lateral pressure, a series of short, controlled, overlapping pull strokes is effected in the coronal direction until all of the calculus is removed *(C)*. When performing pull strokes with Gracey curettes, the part of the shank nearest to the working part must be positioned parallel with the tooth surface; this is an important visual cue to ensure that a correct working angulation is maintained inside the pocket so that the treatment will be as effective as possible.

As a general rule, the scaling stroke is performed by a coordinated movement of the forearm, wrist, and hand that pivots around the finger rest. Although the firm grasp of the fingers around the instrument contributes to the efficacy of the stroke, it must be supported by the strength of the forearm muscles and wrist, thus obtaining maximum power with minimum fatigue.

When the Gracey curette is inserted, the last part of the shank must be oblique to the tooth surface. When the instrument is in position for pull strokes, the last part of the shank must be parallel to the surface of the tooth.

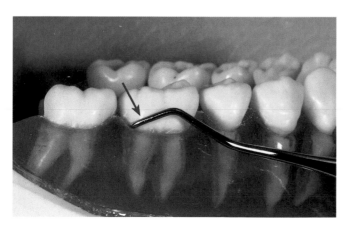

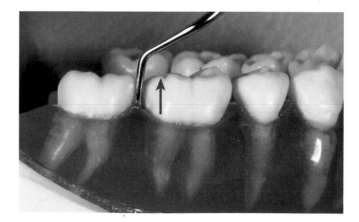

▷ USE OF THE UNIVERSAL CURETTE AND THE SICKLE

Regarding the universal curette and the sickle, it is necessary to consider that both have a facial surface that is perpendicular to the final part of the shank.

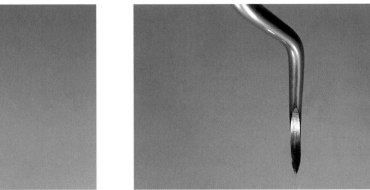

As when utilizing Gracey curettes, the working part of the universal curette or the sickle must be inserted so that the facial surface is as parallel to the tooth surface as possible. Then, tightening the grasp to obtain a firm, secure grip, the working part is opened by moving the final part of the shank away from the tooth until it assumes an angulation that is more than 60 degrees and less than 85 degrees with respect to the tooth surface. However, considering that the facial surface is at 90 degrees with respect to the final part of the shank, the latter must be oblique to the tooth surface when pull strokes are performed to establish the proper working angulation (70 degrees) inside the pocket.

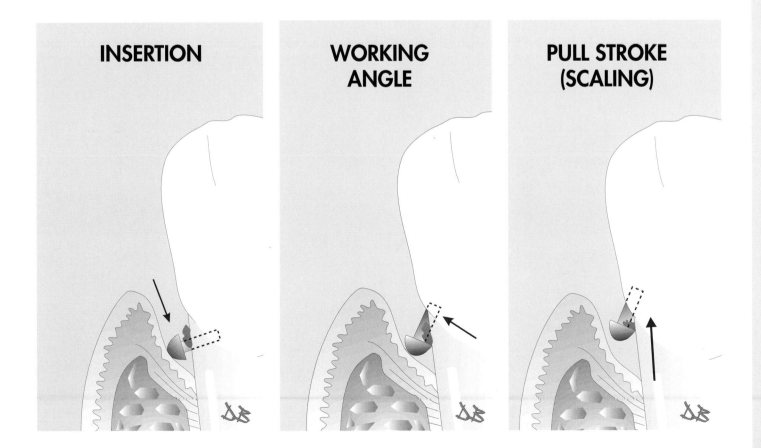

| INSERTION | WORKING ANGLE | PULL STROKE (SCALING) |

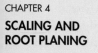
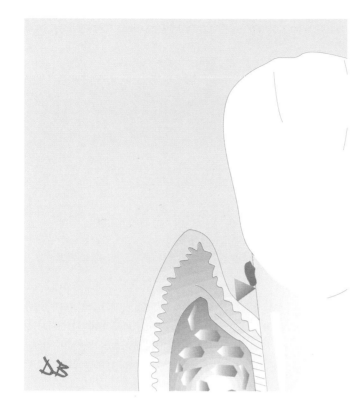

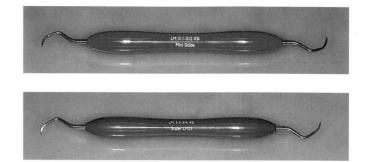

Experience has led me to prefer the sickle for the removal of supragingival calculus and for the treatment of gingivitis and shallow pockets. It is also ideal for cleaning interproximal areas in which there are very narrow spaces. The sickle has two cutting edges, and it is utilized following the same technique used with Gracey curettes 11/12 and 13/14, which have cutting edges located on the same side or on the opposite side with respect to the last bend of the shank.

In fact, the cutting edge of the sickle that is located on the same side as the last bend of the shank is used for treatment of the mesial surfaces, while the one located on the opposite side is used for the distal surfaces. If lateral pressure is applied to the root surfaces during instrumentation, the slightly beveled back of the sickle will not provoke damage to the soft tissue and therefore will not cause the patient any pain.

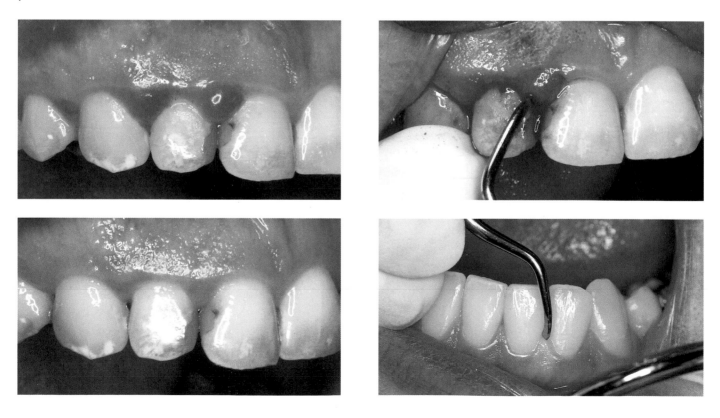

▷ CONSIDERATIONS ON ROOT PLANING

Once the calculus has been removed, the root surfaces are usually planed with curettes to produce smooth root surfaces. Whereas with scaling the deposits of calculus are dislodged from the tooth by fragmenting them with the cutting edge, the proper technique of root planing calls for a delicate movement. Numerous long strokes are performed in various directions that may be vertical, crosswise, and horizontal. This procedure avoids creating nicks and gouges on the roots. After root planing, the root surfaces should feel smooth on probing.

Previously, root planing called for the removal of softened and necrotic cementum in order to render the root surface hard and smooth. In fact, Aleo et al[2] in 1974 assessed the presence and biologic activity of endotoxins on root cementum and affirmed that it is necessary to remove all necrotic cementum because it is laden with bacterial endotoxins. Thus, the indication was to "scrape" the root surface meticulously in order to eliminate the necrotic cementum, that is, the bacterial endotoxins. In fact, the prior goal of this treatment was to establish a "glassy smooth" root surface, which, however, often had the disadvantage of provoking root hypersensitivity.

In contrast, Moore et al[19] in 1986 studied the actual distribution of endotoxins on root surfaces and found that endotoxins only adhere weakly to the surface and are not an integral part of the root surface. Therefore, they concluded that it is not necessary to plane the root of the tooth in depth.

Then, Nyman and coworkers[22,23] in 1986 and 1988 carried out further studies, affirming that it is possible to obtain the same improvement in periodontal health with or without removal of the cementum exposed to disease ("infected" cementum). Therefore, the removal of root cementum aimed at the elimination of eventual endotoxins present in the cementum itself is not necessary in order to obtain periodontal healing.

A study conducted in 1995 by Mombelli et al[18] also confirmed that the deliberate removal of infected cementum is no longer justified. These studies instead evidence that the reduction of the specific subgingival microorganisms responsible for periodontal disease is essential for the success of periodontal treatment. Similar results were also obtained from a study carried out in 1994 by Gmür et al[11] in which plastic curettes were utilized.

The removal of a certain quantity of the cementum cannot be avoided during the removal of calculus. The deliberate removal of cementum to eliminate endotoxins should be avoided. Avoiding the removal of cementum can prevent the onset of root hypersensitivity and the possible penetration of bacteria into the dentin.[1]

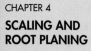
▷ **THE SYNTETTE CURETTE**

I have found a special curette that is very useful in the execution of good root planing: the Syntette (LM Dental).

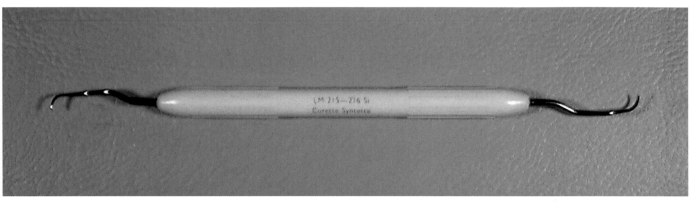

This instrument is a particular type of curette with two cutting edges but with a facial surface that forms a "roof," or rather has both slopes offset at 70 degrees, similar to the Gracey curettes. This special form was designed to permit the operator to work on both mesial and distal surfaces without having to change the curette. However, the advantages that I have found during root planing are not maintained during scaling, when the working part of this curette is too cumbersome, making it difficult for the operator to obtain the sensitivity necessary to perform calculus removal effectively.

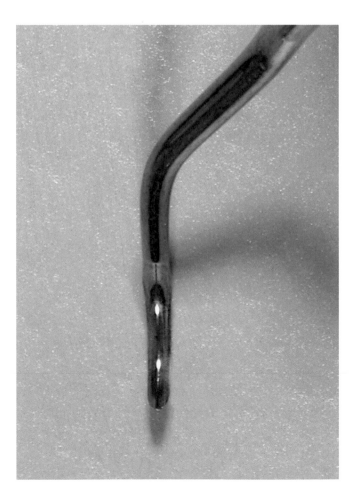

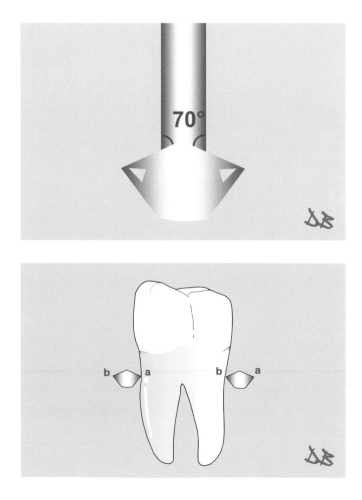

▷ INSTRUMENTS FOR DIFFICULT-TO-REACH AREAS

If the periodontal pockets are not very deep, scaling and root planing can be performed by choosing the most appropriate instruments among Gracey curettes, the sickle, and the Syntette.

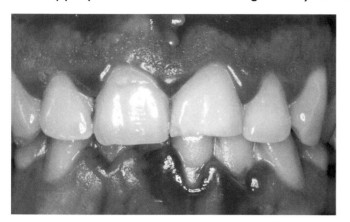

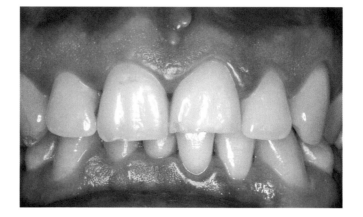

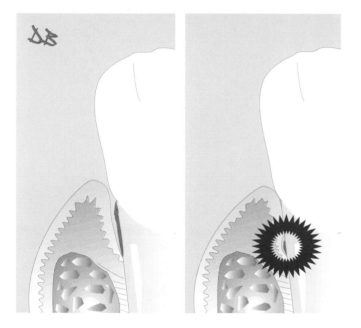

However, other instruments are necessary in order to treat the bottom of very deep periodontal pockets (9 to 10 mm). If traditional instruments were used in this situation, it might not be possible to perform adequate treatment in the deepest part of the pocket, and this might create the risk of a shirt-stud abscess. In order to avoid this risk, and to obtain an excellent state of cleanliness in the deepest and most difficult-to-reach pockets, it is necessary to use instruments that have a longer shank and a thinner, shorter working part. Examples of these types of instruments are Gracey Mini curettes and the Syntette Mini curette (LM Dental).

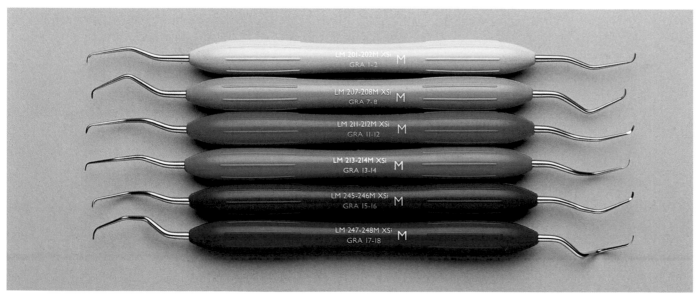

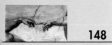
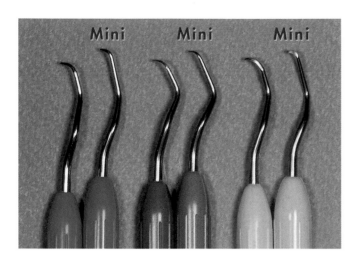

The most widely used Gracey Minis are the 11/12 and the 13/14, which can be supported by the Syntette Mini. These curettes make it possible to perform effective instrumentation in very deep pockets around anterior or posterior teeth.

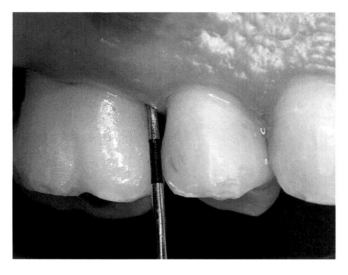

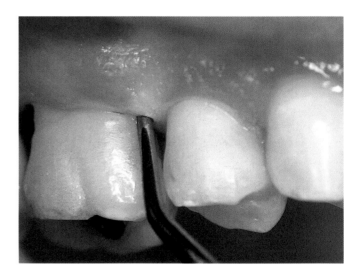

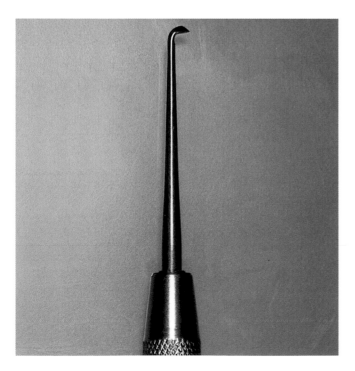

In deep pockets of anterior teeth, a particular type of sickle (No. 00, Produits Dentaires, Switzerland) with a straight shank, a very small working part, and two cutting edges is also extremely useful.

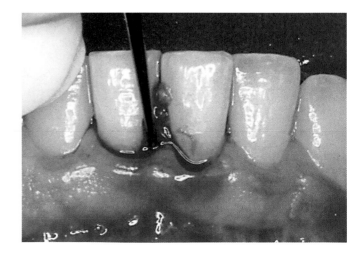

CLINICAL CASE TREATED WITH INSTRUMENTS FOR DIFFICULT-TO-REACH AREAS

Initial Examination
The 35-year-old male patient arrived at the dental surgery for recurring abscesses on tooth 21. The initial examination performed by the dentist detected 11 mm of clinical probing depth and minor periodontal problems at some other areas. The radiograph revealed the presence of a deep, angular bone defect corresponding to the probing depth of 11 mm.

Treatment Planning
The status of hygiene was not satisfactory; therefore, the dentist planned two appointments for treatment to be performed by the hygienist.

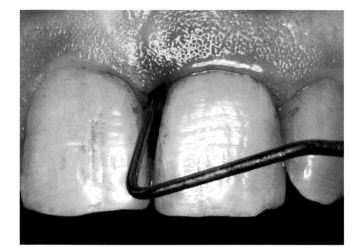
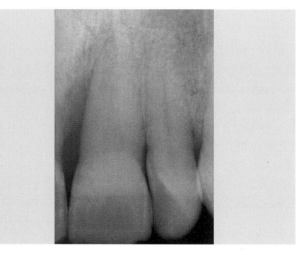

Treatment
During the first oral hygiene appointment, I motivated the patient and gave him the necessary instructions regarding oral hygiene. Because there was only one deep pocket mesial of tooth 21, in a phase of quiescence, I decided to treat it immediately, after the administration of local anesthesia, utilizing Gracey Mini curettes, the PD sickle, and the Amdent ultrasonic instrument. A week later, I treated the other pockets without local anesthesia because they were shallow.

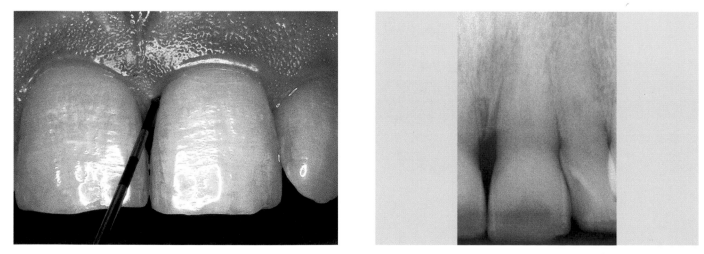

The patient's situation improved, and at reevaluation after 3 months, the deep mesial probing depth proved to be resolved. The radiographic examination 1 year after active treatment showed that the angular bone defect was almost entirely closed.

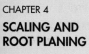

▷ **PROGRAM OF TREATMENT FOR SCALING AND ROOT PLANING**

The first patient visit is conducted by the dentist, who gathers all the information necessary to make a diagnosis and establish a treatment plan, determining at the same time the number of appointments the hygienist will require to perform thorough scaling and root planing. The number of appointments necessary for a patient with severe generalized periodontitis is essentially determined by the number of residual teeth, the depth of the pockets, and the results that the treatment aims to obtain.

During these appointments, the patient is adequately motivated, instructed in the techniques of self-performed oral hygiene, and subjected to periodontal treatment. The first appointment is used to motivate the patient and to teach the correct use of the toothbrush. The others are necessary to perform scaling and root planing, integrated with instructions regarding the use of a suitable interdental instrument and other adjunctive devices that may be necessary.

During each appointment, it is preferable to treat only one quadrant of the mouth thoroughly, performing both supragingival and subgingival scaling. Supragingival gross scaling is called for only in the presence of extensive deposits of calculus that would impede adequate probing and proper oral hygiene procedures. After 3 months, the dentist conducts a careful reevaluation of the condition of the gingiva, the depth of the pockets, tooth mobility, and the patient's plaque control. On the basis of this important analysis, the dentist will decide what further therapy must be performed.

CASE PRESENTATION

Initial Examination
The 63-year-old male patient arrived at the dental surgery worried about the fact that some of his teeth showed signs of mobility. His case history showed that he was in good health. The clinical examination and radiographs revealed the presence of severe generalized adult periodontitis.

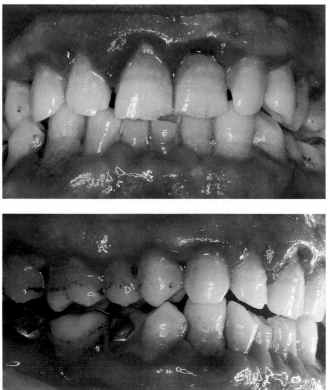

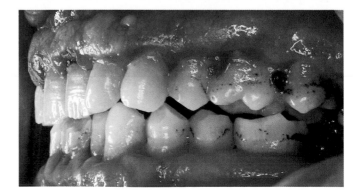

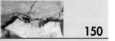

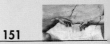

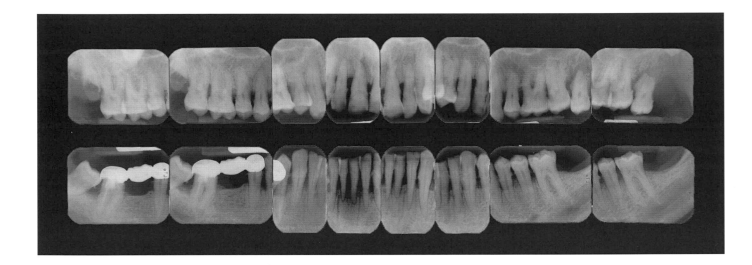

Treatment Planning

The dentist decided to extract the third molars and planned five nonsurgical treatment appointments to be performed by the hygienist. Prior to these treatments, the dentist would administer local anesthesia.

Treatment

During the first oral hygiene appointment, I motivated the patient and gave him the necessary instructions regarding oral hygiene. In the course of the next four appointments, after the dentist had administered local anesthesia, I treated each quadrant using Gracey curettes, Gracey Mini curettes, PD sickle, and the Amdent ultrasonic instrument.

Reevaluation

Three months after the end of the cause-related therapy, the results obtained were evaluated. These results revealed that the patient's collaboration was fairly good, but not excellent. The periodontal situation was noticeably improved in the maxilla, while the situation in the mandible required further treatment.

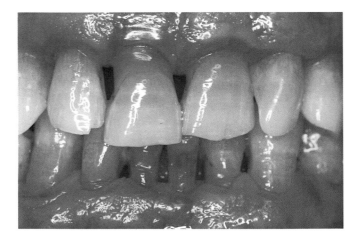

REEVALUATION — R.G. 63

Tooth	m	b	d	l	Furc Inv	Mob	Tooth	m	b	d	l	Furc Inv	Mob
18							48	6*	*	*	*		
17							47		6*				
16					B1		46						
15							45	6*					
14							44			6*	4*		1
13							43						
12							42	5*					
11		5*	5*			1	41				5*		1
21							31	4			5*		1
22							32	4			4		
23							33	4			4		
24							34						
25							35						
26							36						
27						1	37						
28							38						

PI 35%   GBI 30%   BOP 13%

After the dentist's reevaluation, I re-treated, nonsurgically and under local anesthesia, all residual bleeding pockets. After this appointment, the dentist performed the necessary endodontic and restorative therapies.

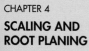

Recall

At the recall after 3 more months, the results were positive. The pathologic pockets had practically disappeared, and despite the presence of plaque in some sites, the tooth mobility had noticeably decreased. The patient was very satisfied, showing an evident motivation and the capacity to understand how to maintain an optimal status of periodontal health.

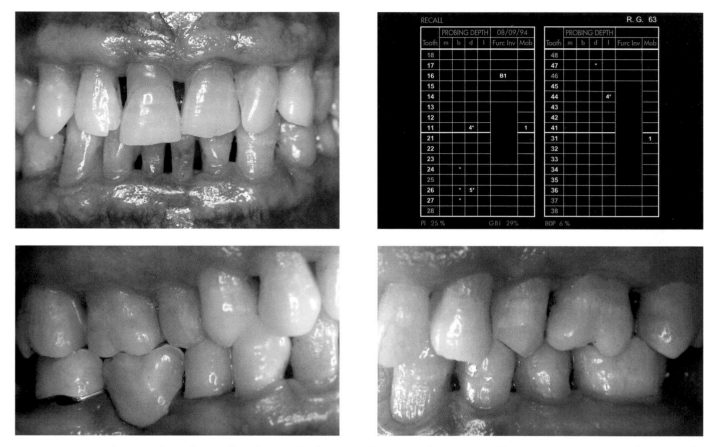

RECALL   R. G. 63

	PROBING DEPTH				08/09/94			PROBING DEPTH					
Tooth	m	b	d	l	Furc Inv	Mob	Tooth	m	b	d	l	Furc Inv	Mob
18							48						
17							47		.				
16					B1		46						
15							45						
14							44				4*		
13							43						
12							42						
11		4*				1	41						
21							31						1
22							32						
23							33						
24	.						34						
25							35						
26	.	5*					36						
27	.						37						
28							38						

PI 25 %   GBI 29%   BOP 6 %

The 4-year radiographs taken after the end of active therapy show a stable situation. Punctual at recalls every 3 to 4 months, the patient has maintained this situation.

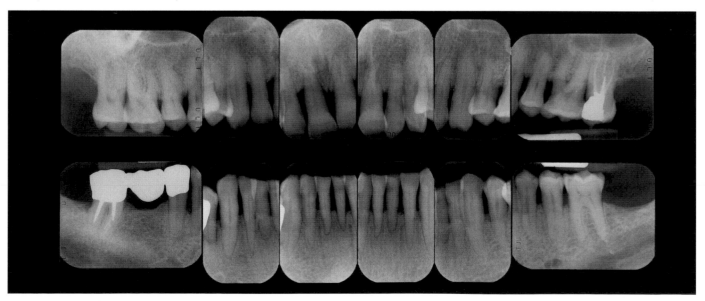

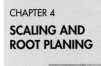
▶ ROTATING INSTRUMENTS

When scaling and root planing have been completed, it is useful to polish the tooth surfaces and eliminate any eventual extrinsic dental stains. This discoloration on the tooth surfaces is evident if oral hygiene procedures have not been strictly observed. Once removed, these stains tend to reform and may then be removed by means of scaling and tooth polishing. These stains are caused by external agents and are classified according to their origin and distinguished according to their color. The stains may be of the following origins:

1. Bacterial: yellow, green, black, orange (chromogenic bacteria)

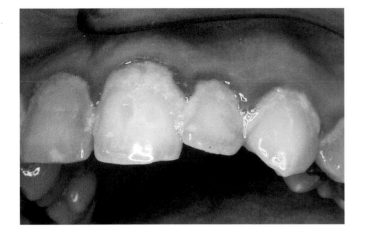
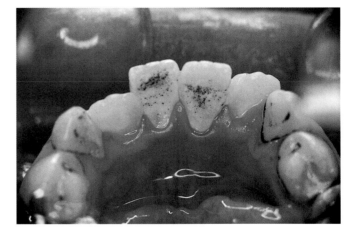

2. Alimentary and nicotine: black/brown (tea, coffee, licorice, spices, tobacco)

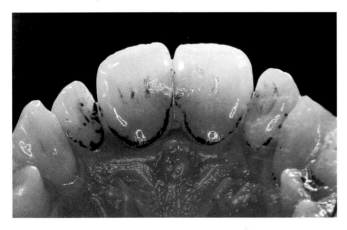
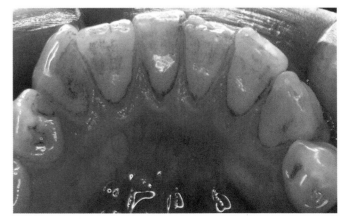

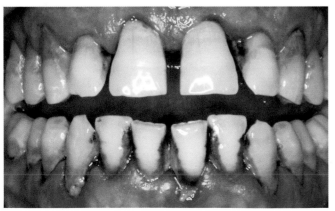
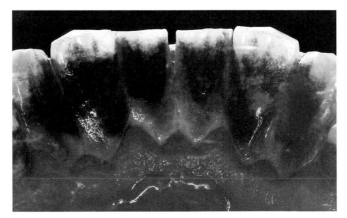

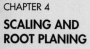
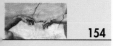
3. Chemical: black/brown (chlorhexidine)

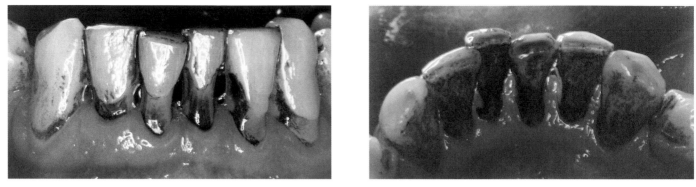

Dental polishing includes all of the procedures aimed at the removal of extrinsic stains from the dentition and the establishment of perfectly clean and smooth tooth surfaces. These stains may be eliminated with the curette and the sickle. A handpiece may also be utilized; in this case, a rubber cup or bristle brush is inserted into the tip. Both of these devices can be used with polishing paste, which may have different degrees of abrasiveness (eg, Proxyt, Vivacare, Liechtenstein). A high RDA is useful when tenacious stains are present, while a low RDA is necessary when teeth are sensitive.

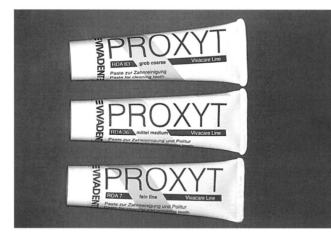

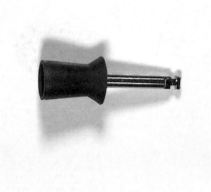

Rotating instruments are used in the following manner. The handpiece is grasped and the rubber cup is dipped into the abrasive paste. A finger rest is also necessary in this case. The rubber cup is applied to the tooth surface, starting near the gingival margin, and the rotation follows the external form of the tooth. Polishing must be performed at a low speed to limit the amount of heat produced. If the bristle brush is used, it is not advisable to work near the gingival margin to avoid injury to the gingiva.

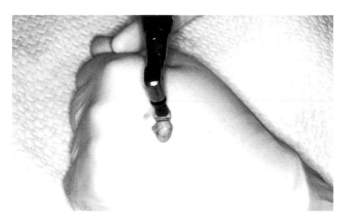

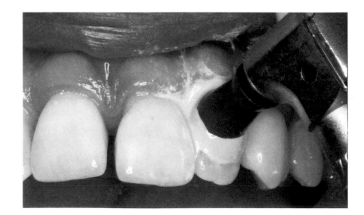

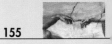

A cone-shaped cup is best suited for wide interdental spaces.

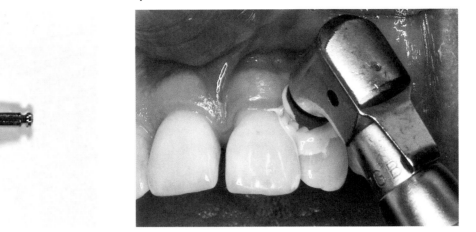

Finishing strips with only one abrasive side composed of two different grains (Hawe Neos Dental, Switzerland) are the best choice for narrow interdental spaces.

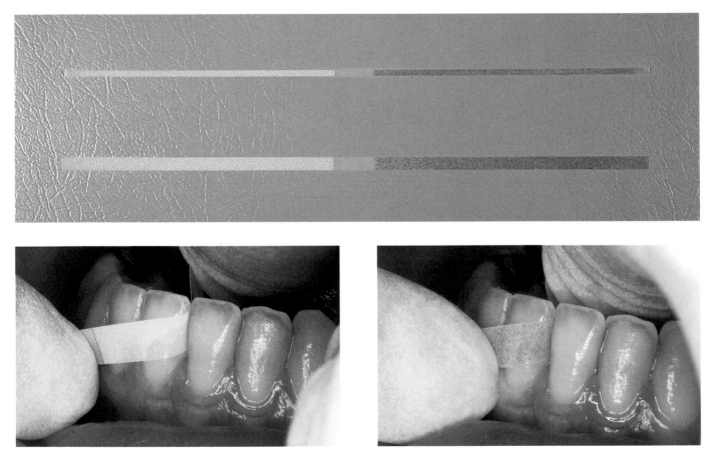

As an alternative to the polishing methods illustrated, many operators use a pressure jet, composed of sodium bicarbonate and water, directed at the tooth (eg, Prophy-Jet, Dentsply). This jet should be used only with the concomitant support of a good aspirating device; otherwise, a veil of dust might cover the patient, the operator, and the furnishings. This method is not recommended for use on hypersensitive teeth or in areas with gingival recessions.

▶ **TABLE OF REFERENCE**

The following table facilitates the choice of the most appropriate instrument for supragingival and subgingival scaling in relation to various clinical probing depths.

CLINICAL SITUATION	INSTRUMENTS
GINGIVITIS	• Ultrasonic or sonic device chosen in relation to the quantity of calculus present on the tooth surfaces • Sickle for the mesial, distal, buccal, and lingual surfaces • Syntette curette for root planing of necks • Handpiece with rubber cup or brush and polishing paste • Abrasive strips for narrow interdental spaces
PERIODONTITIS WITH POCKETS ≤ 7 MM	• Ultrasonic or sonic device chosen in relation to the quantity of calculus present on the tooth surfaces • Sickle for pockets up to 4 mm • Gracey Curettes: 5/6 for surfaces of anterior teeth 7/8 for buccal and lingual surfaces of premolars and molars 11/12 for mesial surfaces premolars and molars 13/14 distal surfaces of premolars and molars 15/16 for mesial surfaces of molars (shank with more acutely angled bends) 17/18 for distal surfaces of molars (shank with more acutely angled bends) • Syntette curette for root planing • Handpiece with rubber cup or brush and polishing paste
PERIODONTITIS WITH POCKETS > 7 MM	• Ultrasonic or sonic device chosen in relation to the quantity of calculus present on the tooth surfaces • Gracey Mini curettes 11/12, 13/14 chosen in relation to the surfaces to be treated (as indicated above) • PD sickle No. 00 for anterior teeth • Syntette curette Mini for root planing • Handpiece with rubber cup or brush and polishing paste

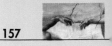
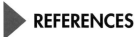 **REFERENCES**

1. Adriaens PA, De Boever JA, Loeche WJ. Bacteria invasion in root cementum and radicular dentin of periodontally diseased teeth in humans. J Periodontol 1988;59:222–230.

2. Aleo J, De Renzis F, Farber PA, Varboncoeur AP. The presence and biologic activity of cementum-bound endotoxin. J Periodontol 1974;45:672–675.

3. Axelsson P, Lindhe J. Effect of controlled oral hygiene procedures on caries and periodontal disease in adults. J Clin Periodontol 1978;5:133–151.

4. Badersten A, Nilvéus R, Egelberg J. Effect of nonsurgical periodontal therapy. I. Moderately advanced periodontitis. J Clin Periodontol 1981;8:57–72.

5. Badersten A, Nilvéus R, Egelberg J. Effect of nonsurgical periodontal therapy. II. Severely advanced periodontitis. J Clin Periodontol 1984;11:63–76.

6. Badersten A, Nilvéus R, Egelberg J. Effect of nonsurgical periodontal therapy. III. Single versus repeated instrumentation. J Clin Periodontol 1984;11:114–124.

7. Badersten A, Nilvéus R, Egelberg J. Effect of non-surgical periodontal therapy (IV). Operator variability. J Clin Periodontol 1985;12:190–200.

8. Björn H, Lindhe J. The influence of periodontal instruments on the tooth surface. A methodological study. Odontol Revy 1962;13:355–369.

9. Carranza FA Jr. Glickman's Clinical Periodontology, ed 7. chapters 40, 41, 42. Philadelphia: W.B. Saunders, 1990:chap 40–42.

10. Cercek JF, Kiger RD, Garrett S, Egelberg J. Relative effects of plaque control and instrumentation on the clinical parameters of human periodontal disease. J Clin Periodontol 1983;10:46–56.

11. Gmür R, Saxer UP, Guggenheim B. Effects of blunt scaling on periodontal status and subgingival microorganisms. A pilot study. Schweiz Monatsschr Zahnmed 1994;104:430–439.

12. Hämmerle CHF, Joss A, Lang NP. Short-term effects of initial periodontal therapy (hygienic phase). J Clin Periodontol 1991;18:233–239.

13. Hellewege KD. La Levigatura Radicolare. Milano: Scienza e Tecnica Dentistica Edizioni Internazionali, 1988:chap 3.

14. Leon EL, Vogel RI. A comparison of the effectiveness of hand scaling and ultrasonic debridement in furcations as evaluated by differential dark-field microscopy. J Periodontol 1987;58:86–94.

15. Lindhe J. Clinical Periodontology and Implant Dentistry, ed 3. Copenhagen: Munksgaard, 1997:chap 15.

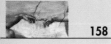
16. Loos B, Nylund K, Claffey N, Egelberg J. Clinical effects of root debridement in molar and non-molar teeth: A 2-year follow-up. J Clin Periodontol 1989;16:498–504.

17. Lovdal A, Arno A, Schei O, Waerhaug J. Combined effect of subgingival scaling and root planing and controlled oral hygiene on the incidence of gingivitis. Acta Odontol Scand 1961;19:537–555.

18. Mombelli A, Nyman S, Brägger U, Wennström J, Lang NP. Clinical and microbiological changes associated with an altered subgingival environment induced by periodontal pocket reduction. J Clin Periodontol 1995;22:780–787.

19. Moore J, Wilson M, Kieser JB. The distribution of bacterial lipopolysaccharide (endotoxin) in relation to periodontally involved root surfaces. J Clin Periodontol 1986;13:748–751.

20. Morrison EC, Ramfjörd SP, Hill RW. Short-term effects of initial, nonsurgical periodontal treatment (hygienic phase). J Clin Periodontol 1980;7:199–211.

21. Nordland P, Garrett S, Kiger R, Vanooteghem R, Hutchens LH, Egelberg J. The effect of plaque control and root debridement in molar teeth. J Clin Periodontol 1987;14:231–236.

22. Nyman S, Sarhed G, Ericsson I, Gottlow J, Karring T. Role of "diseased" root cementum in healing following treatment of periodontal disease. An experimental study in the dog. J Periodontal Res 1986;21:496–503.

23. Nyman S, Westfelt E, Sarhed G, Karring T. Role of "diseased" root cementum in healing following treatment of periodontal disease. A clinical study. J Clin Periodontol 1988;15:464–468.

24. Pattison GL, Pattison AM. Periodontal Instrumentation, ed 2, module III. Norwalk, Conn: Appleton & Lange, 1992.

25. Phagan-Schostok PA, Maloney KL. Igiene Dentale: Attività Clinica Contemporanea. Vol 1: Manuale Clinico. Milano: Scienza e Tecnica Dentistica Edizioni Internazionali, 1992.

26. Proye M, Caton J, Polson A. Initial healing of periodontal pockets after a single episode of root planing monitored by controlled probing forces. J Periodontol 1982;53:296–301.

27. Suomi JD, Green JC, Vermillion JR, Doyle J, Chang JJ, Leatherwood EC. The effect of controlled oral hygiene procedures on the progression of periodontal disease in adults. Results after third and final year. J Periodontol 1971;42:152–160.

28. Torafson T, Kiger R, Selvig KA, Egelberg J. Clinical improvement of gingival conditions following ultrasonic versus hand instrumentation of periodontal pockets. J Clin Periodontol 1979;6:165–176.

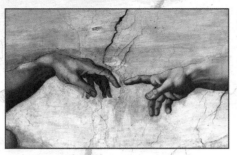

CHAPTER 5

▶ **INSTRUMENT SHARPENING**

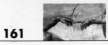
▶ GOAL OF SHARPENING

The efficacy of good instrumentation does not only depend on the operator's skill, but also on the quality of the instrument in use. Therefore, in order to perform effective scaling, all hand instruments must have sharp edges. This ensures that supragingival and subgingival treatment is efficient and precise, and that deposits can be removed from the tooth surfaces with a limited number of strokes.[1,2,4,5]

When curettes are sharp, they have acutely angled cutting edges with a 70-degree angulation.

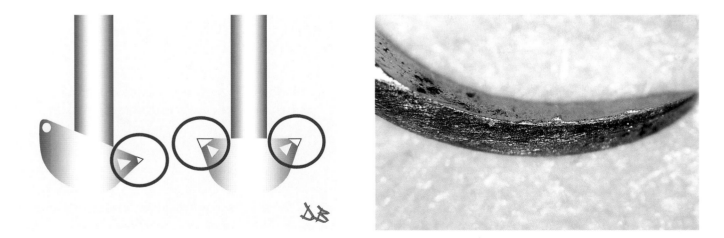

On the other hand, dull curettes have blunt cutting edges with no acute angle and are no longer able to exert a firm grip on the deposits of calculus. In order to perform effective scaling using a curette with dull edges, it is necessary to press the instrument against the root surface harder than with a sharp instrument, thus increasing the working time and physical effort required and provoking the risk of slipping on the calculus and burnishing it rather than managing to remove it. The impression that the root surfaces are smooth is caused by this improper instrumentation.[1,2,4,5]

Sharpening an instrument adequately means restoring its cutting edges while conserving its original form and prolonging its durability.[3]

Instrument sharpening can be performed by hand using sharpening stones (eg, gray Arkansas stone, rust-brown India stone). These stones are abrasive and granulous and are modeled into various shapes and sizes. The choice of the shape of the stone depends on the instrument to be sharpened.

During sharpening, there must be a sufficient source of light in the working area and good stability of the stone and the instrument. Furthermore, the stone must be sterile if it is used during a treatment appointment, because the instruments are then used immediately in the patient's oral cavity.

Sharpening stones may be used in two ways: either the stone is held firm while the working part of the instrument is stroked upon it, or the stone is moved against the working part of the instrument, which is held stationary.

Experience has led me to prefer the flat stone (Arkansas or India) and the cylindric one (Arkansas); as for sharpening, I prefer the technique in which the sharpening stone is held firm while the working part of the instrument is moved upon it.

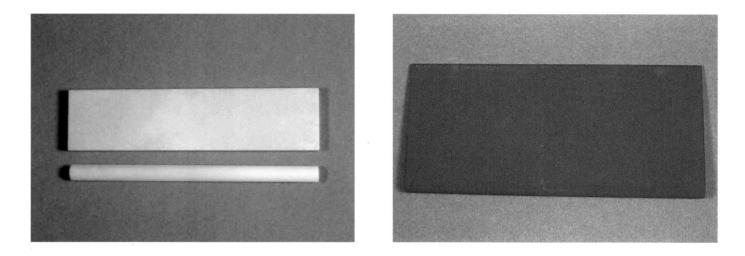

Instruments may be sharpened effectively by applying either the lateral surface or the facial surface of the working part to the stone. Whichever method is chosen, it is always necessary to understand the form and features of each instrument in order to sharpen it adequately.

Different sharpening techniques make it possible to obtain sharp cutting edges. However, many methods call for a series of recommendations that cannot be visualized during the sharpening process, and not all methods completely preserve the original features of the instruments. I believe that the methods of sharpening described below are very easy to learn and considerably simplify the required procedures.

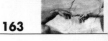

▶ SHARPENING OF THE LATERAL SURFACE

This technique requires a flat sharpening stone and is useful for sharpening both Gracey and Syntette curettes. In both cases, the lateral surface of the working part is applied to the stone.

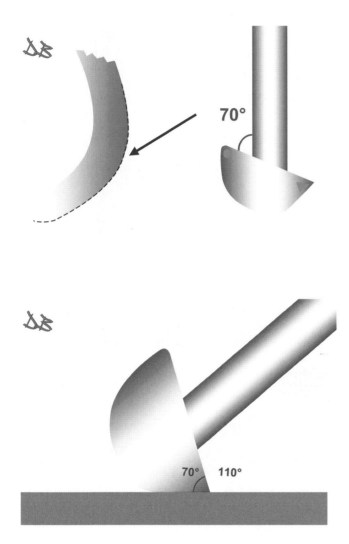

In order to sharpen a Gracey, it is necessary to be very familiar with its shape (see Chapter 4) and to bear in mind the following features:

- The working part of a Gracey is curved.

- Each working part of the Gracey is "offset" at 70 degrees with respect to the last part of the shank.

- The blade has only one cutting edge, which is always the lower one.

- The cutting angle between the facial and lateral surface of the curette is 70 degrees; this means that, when the working part is applied to the stone, the angle between the facial surface and the surface of the stone must be of 110 degrees.

These peculiar features of the Gracey make it impossible to effect frontal sharpening because there is only one edge to sharpen.

It is not easy to see when the facial surface of the blade forms a 110-degree angle with the stone. However, if simple geometric reasoning is applied, it is easy to understand how the last part of the shank must be inclined with respect to the stone: Having the various 70-degree angles as fixed data, and considering that the sum of the internal angles of a triangle is 180 degrees, it is possible to deduce that the angle between the last part of the shank and the stone must be of 40 degrees, that is, about half of a right angle. This inclination is easier to visualize during sharpening.

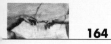
After these very important considerations, the technique for lateral surface sharpening is performed as follows:

1. The instrument is held with a modified pen grasp.
2. The edge to be sharpened is identified.
3. The ring finger and the little finger of the hand that grasps the instrument are placed on the edge of the stone.
4. The lateral surface, located directly under the cutting edge to be sharpened, is applied to the stone.

It will be evident that the last part of the shank automatically forms a 40-degree angle with the stone, confirming that the geometrical reasoning, previously explained, is exact.

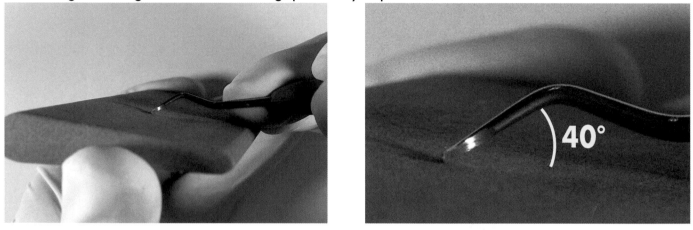

Furthermore, only a part of the lateral surface is in contact with the stone since the working part of the instrument is curved.

After checking to see that the lateral surface has been correctly applied to the stone, it is necessary to move the entire extension of the lateral surface, oscillating it with short movements from the extremity of the shank to the toe, and vice versa, as if it were a pendulum. By keeping the lateral surface of the Gracey continuously in contact with the stone and performing these short, slow, and regular strokes, the cutting edge will be sharpened, automatically and uniformly.

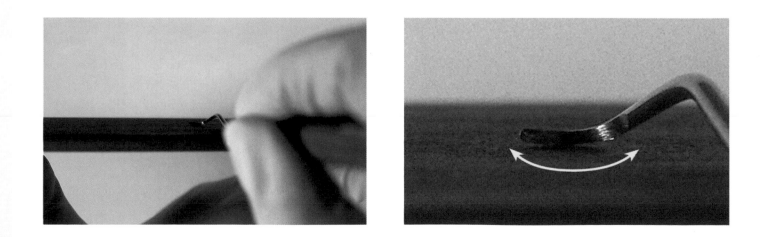

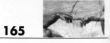

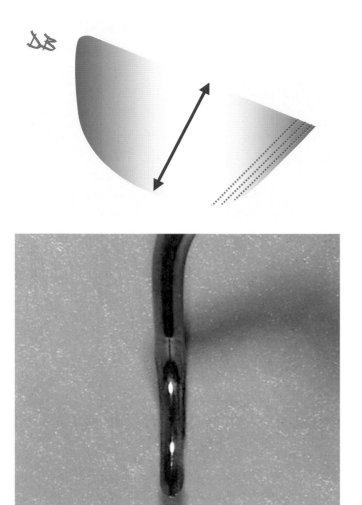

This method of sharpening limits excessive wear of the instrument, which therefore remains resistant because it narrows in width but is not reduced in thickness. In this way it is possible to maintain the original design of Gracey curettes for many months.

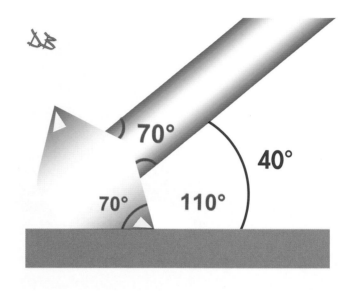

The same technique is also effective for sharpening Syntette curettes, but the procedure must be slightly modified because only the final part of the blade near the tip is curved, while the remaining part rests evenly on the stone. It is therefore necessary to perform two types of movement, maintaining an angle of 40 degrees between the final part of the shank and the surface of the stone:

1. The final part, near the tip, is sharpened with the same procedure described for Gracey curettes: The lateral surface is placed on the stone, and short oscillating movements are performed.
2. The rest of the working part is sharpened by placing the lateral surface on the stone and performing short, straight pull strokes in one direction, thus making it possible to sharpen the entire extension of this part of the blade uniformly.

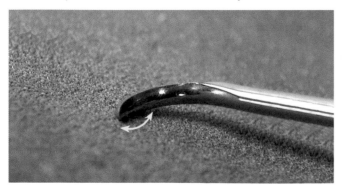

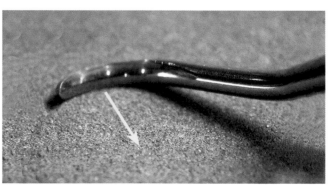

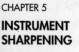
SHARPENING OF THE FACIAL SURFACE

This process, which requires a handheld cylindric stone, is the method that I personally find most effective when sharpening M23, Mini, or LM23 sickles.

The facial surface of the working part is applied to the sharpening stone, when this technique is used.

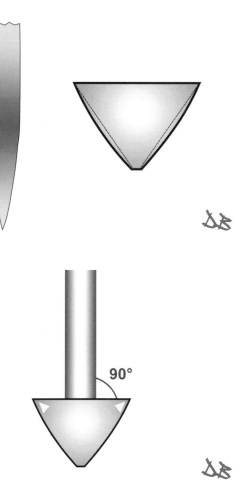

In this case as well, it is necessary to remember the features of sickles:

• The working part of the sickle is straight.

• The lateral surfaces are not flat but slightly curved.

• The facial surface forms a 90-degree angle with the last part of the shank.

• There are two cutting edges to be sharpened at each extremity.

These particular aspects of the sickle make it preferable to sharpen the face of the blade because lateral sharpening would only sharpen one blade at a time and it would be more difficult to conserve the slight curve of the lateral surfaces. Sharpening of the facial surface is less time-consuming, and I consider it the best method to preserve the original features of the instrument.

After these important considerations, the technique of frontal sharpening is performed as follows:

1. The instrument is held in a palm grasp with the fingers turned downward.
2. The two extremities of the cylindric stone are held between the thumb and forefinger of the other hand.

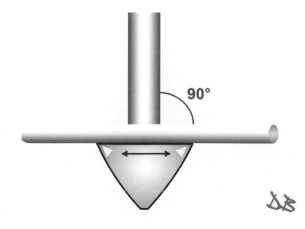

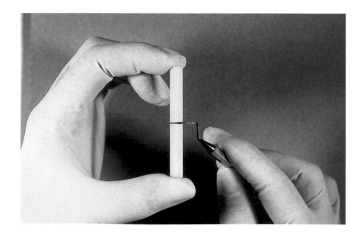

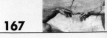
3. The facial surface, where the cutting edges are located, is applied to the stone; the entire length of the facial surface must be evenly in contact with the stone, and the last part of the shank must form a 90-degree angle with the surface of the stone.

4. After having correctly positioned the facial surface, the blade is moved upon the stone, sliding the facial surface itself back and forth.

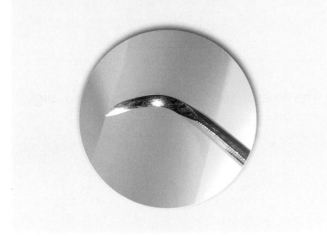

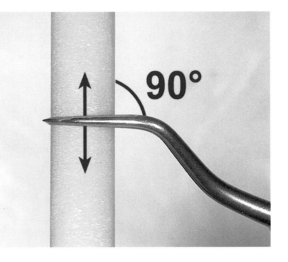

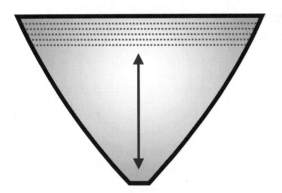

This easy and rapid method of sharpening makes it possible to sharpen the two cutting edges of each working part simultaneously and uniformly. However, the disadvantage is that this procedure rapidly wears down the thickness of the working part, the resistance of which depends on its thickness, not on its width. In spite of this drawback, I have noticed that sickles sharpened with this technique always maintain their original form and can be used for many months, because only a minimum quantity of material is removed each time they are sharpened.

This easy technique may also be used to sharpen universal curettes properly.

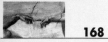
Frontal sharpening is used to sharpen PD sickles because it is necessary to take into account the fact that the facial surface of a PD sickle forms a right angle with the shank; therefore, this surface must be applied to the edge of the flat stone in order to restore the right angle.

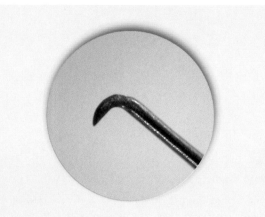

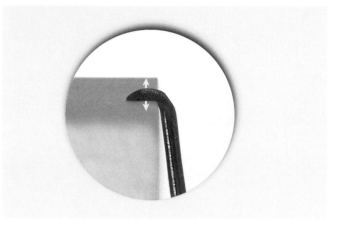

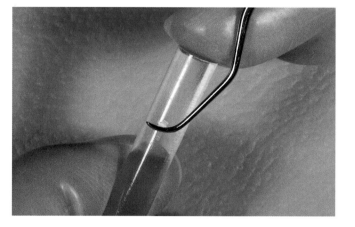

Sharpness can be evaluated by adapting the instrument against a plastic testing stick. This test is usually performed during the phase in which one is learning the techniques of sharpening; generally, it is no longer necessary once the operator has acquired experience.

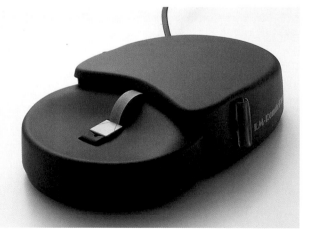

The market now offers various devices that may be useful in sharpening curettes and sickles; however, their initial cost is usually quite high. Among these, I have had the opportunity to use and to appreciate LM Rondo (LM Dental), whose mechanical structure and design make it possible to sharpen instruments properly, while maintaining their original features.

On the basis of their own manual dexterity, operators may choose the techniques for sharpening that they individually prefer, provided that the general goals of the procedure are always maintained. My advice, however, is to try to sharpen instruments using the manual methods described in this chapter, which have always given good results.

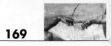

▶ TABLE OF REFERENCE

The following table facilitates the choice of the most appropriate method of sharpening in relation to the various instruments to be sharpened.

SURFACE	METHOD

LATERAL SURFACE

GRACEY CURETTE

- Apply the lateral surface of the curette to the flat stone.
- Form a 40-degree angle between the last part of the shank and the surface of the stone.
- Oscillate the entire extension of the working part, from the extremity of the shank toward the tip and vice versa.

SYNTETTE CURETTE

- Apply the lateral surface of the curette to the flat stone.
- Form a 40-degree angle between the last part of the shank and the surface of the stone.
- Oscillate the tip of the working part.
- Sharpen the rest of the working part with short, straight pull strokes in only one direction.

FACIAL SURFACE

M23 SICKLE
LM23 SICKLE
MINI SICKLE
UNIVERSAL CURETTE

- Apply the facial surface of the instrument to the cylindrical stone.
- Form a 90-degree angle between the last part of the shank and the surface of the stone.
- Move the blade on the stone, sliding it back and forth.

PD SICKLE

- Place the facial surface of the instrument on the edge of the flat stone.
- Move the blade on the stone, sliding it back and forth.

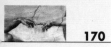
▶ REFERENCES

1. Carranza FA Jr. Glickman's Clinical Periodontology, ed 7. Philadelphia: W.B. Saunders, 1990:chap 43.

2. Hellewege KD. La Levigatura Radicocare. Milano: Scienza e Tecnica Dentistica Edizioni Internazionali, 1988:chap 4.

3. Paquette OE, Levin MP. The sharpening of scaling instruments: I. An examination of principles. J Periodontol 1977;48:163–168.

4. Pattison GL, Pattison AM. Periodontal Instrumentation, ed 2, module IV. Norwalk, Conn: Appleton & Lange, 1992.

5. Phagan-Schostok PA, Maloney KL. Igiene Dentale: Attività Clinica Contemporanea. Vol. 1: Manuale Clinico, unità 13. Milano: Scienza e Tecnica Dentistica Edizioni Internazionali, 1992.

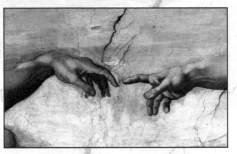

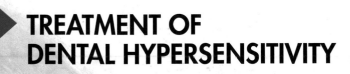

CHAPTER 6

▶ TREATMENT OF
DENTAL HYPERSENSITIVITY

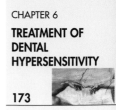
Dental hypersensitivity is a condition that may set in when exposed dentin is exceptionally sensitive to:

- Thermal stimuli (hot or cold)
- Chemical stimuli (acidic foods)
- Mechanical stimuli (toothbrushing, root planing)

Dental hypersensitivity is a common problem among patients with dental abrasions or gingival recessions. Furthermore, patients often complain of increased sensitivity after periodontal treatment, because not only plaque and calculus but also cementum and superficial parts of the dentin are removed from the root surfaces, thus exposing the dentinal tubules, which consequently become sensitive to the stimuli that come from the oral cavity, causing root hypersensitivity.[1,7]

Although the exact mechanism has not been defined yet, it is known that external stimuli cause sudden movements of fluid in the exposed dentinal tubules,[3] thus eliciting activation of the nerve fibers that induce pain. The painful symptoms may vary in duration and intensity. They are frequently acute immediately after periodontal treatment, but the pain is usually transitory and subsides or disappears after a few weeks as a result of the natural occlusion of the exposed dentinal tubules.[9]

Sometimes, however, this may become a chronic condition because the dentinal tubules in certain areas remain open to the extent that the slightest contact between the toothbrush and the surface of the root dentin may cause intense pain. This condition must be given due consideration because it is very unpleasant and also compromises correct oral hygiene procedures.

Acidic foods, such as fruit juices, yogurt, and wine, have been implicated as a cause of hypersensitivity.[2] Because of their acidity and potential to etch the dentin, they can dissolve the natural occlusions of the dentinal tubules or prevent their formation. Therefore, it is important to inquire about patients' dietary habits to verify if their hypersensitivity may be caused by overconsumption of citrus fruit, green fruit, apples, or any other acidic food or beverage.[7]

Plaque control is, however, of essential importance in the treatment of root hypersensitivity. In fact, clinical tests have shown that over the course of time, meticulous oral hygiene measures favor the development of smooth, hard root surfaces that are not sensitive because the dentinal tubules are occluded.[5]

On the other hand, when acute symptoms of root hypersensitivity are present, it is difficult for the patient to maintain the level of plaque control necessary to favor the natural occlusion of the dentinal tubules. It is therefore necessary to introduce a specific therapy by applying substances that have the potential to seal the tubular openings, thus making the pain subside as rapidly as possible and guaranteeing patients a more comfortable condition that enables them to carry out self-performed plaque control more adequately.[7]

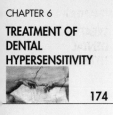
In recent years, a wide variety of therapeutic agents have been proposed. There are specific products for professional application and also for home care. These products are composed of chemical agents that have the potential to seal the openings of the dentinal tubules, thus eliminating the possibility of rapid movements of fluids within the tubules. Examples of such chemical agents are strontium chloride, sodium monofluorophosphate, sodium fluoride, calcium hypophosphate, calcium hydroxide, potassium nitrate, potassium oxalate, glutaraldehyde, and stannous fluoride.

Unfortunately, the results obtained with the currently existing methods are not always predictable.[8] These therapeutic techniques do not always determine a definitive occlusion of the dentinal tubules; nevertheless, they do make it temporarily possible for the patient to perform correct oral hygiene procedures, which favor the natural occlusion of the dentinal tubules.

▶ PROFESSIONAL APPLICATION

Among the many desensitizing agents having the potential to repair and close the dentinal tubules, the following are the ones I prefer for topical applications performed in the dental office:

- Potassium oxalate
- Sodium fluoride 2.26%
- Calcium hydroxide

▷ POTASSIUM OXALATE

Potassium oxalate (eg, Protect, Butler, Chicago, IL) is available in single-dose vials, from which the liquid is delivered to a cotton pellet situated at one end.

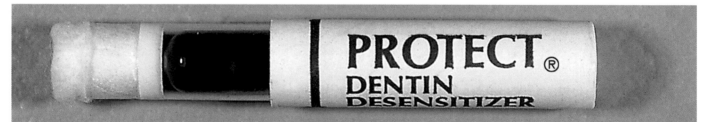

Potassium oxalate is also available in bottles, from which the necessary dose is poured into a small cup. A little sponge is then dipped into the liquid and used for local application of the product.

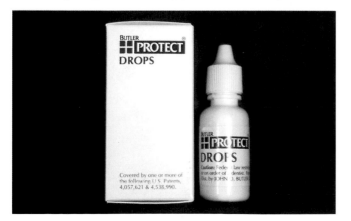

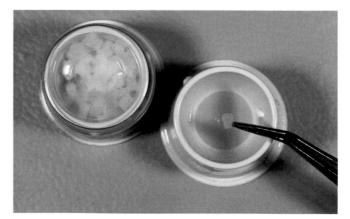

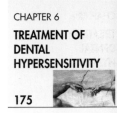

Once the sensitive surface of the tooth has been adequately polished and dried, Protect is dabbed on the area in question and left in place for at least 2 minutes.

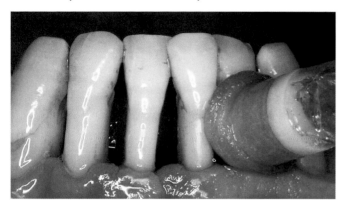
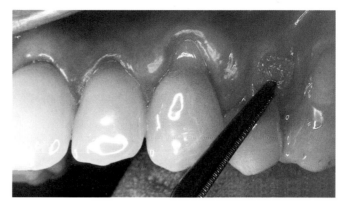

After rinsing with water, air stimulation by means of the air syringe is used to reevaluate the symptoms of hypersensitivity. If necessary, it is possible to repeat the treatment immediately or during the next appointments.

▷ SODIUM FLUORIDE 2.26%

Duraphat is a sodium fluoride varnish available in a tube.

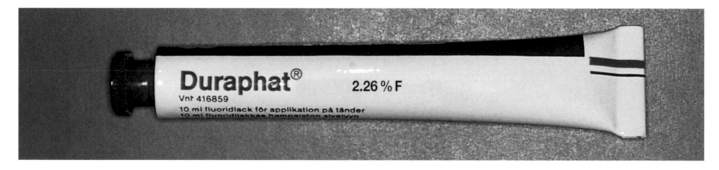

A small quantity of varnish is placed on the back of a gloved hand. After the tooth surfaces are thoroughly polished and dried, the varnish is applied to the sensitive surface by means of a small brush.

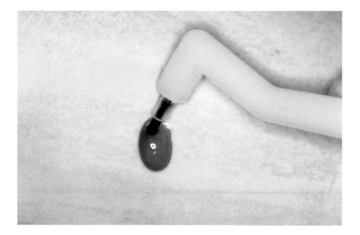
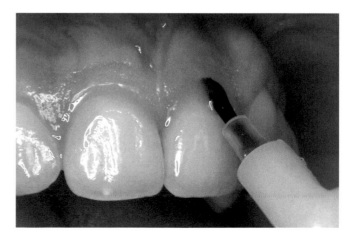

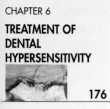
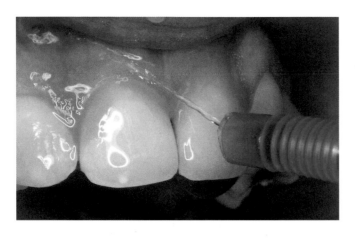

The varnish is then fixed on the tooth surfaces with a fine stream of water trickled from the syringe of the dental unit.

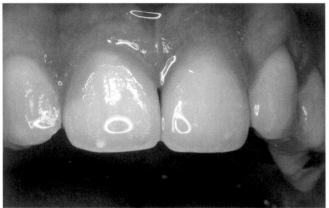

After treatment, the patient must not smoke or eat solid foods for at least 4 hours. The varnish must remain in contact with the tooth surface for 24 hours, during which the patient must not perform any type of oral hygiene procedures in the treated area.

Duraphat is also available in vials that may be inserted into a syringe that is normally used for local anesthesia. The product is then applied through a needle with a blunt point and a diameter large enough to permit the passage of the varnish.

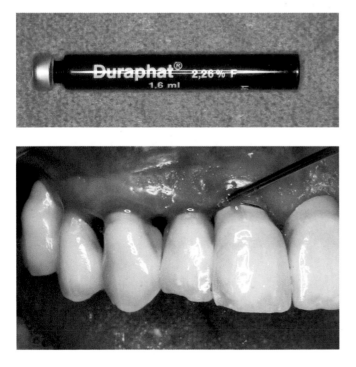

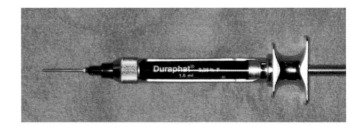

Use of the syringe is very convenient when it is necessary to apply this varnish on many tooth surfaces. It is also useful in the treatment of patients who are susceptible to caries and in maintenance therapy to prevent caries on abutment teeth supporting prostheses.

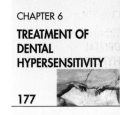
▷ CALCIUM HYDROXIDE

Calcium hydroxide (eg, Calxyl, Oco Präparate, Germany) is placed in a small cup and then mixed with physiologic saline solution until a dense paste is obtained. After the sensitive tooth surfaces are polished and dried, the paste is dabbed on these surfaces utilizing a small sponge.

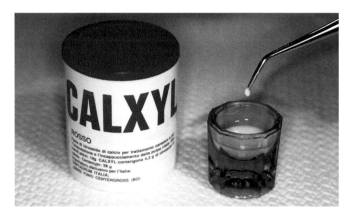
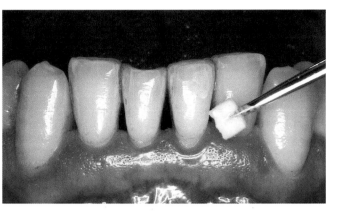

The product is left in place, and the area is protected with a periodontal dressing, which the patient removes after 2 days.

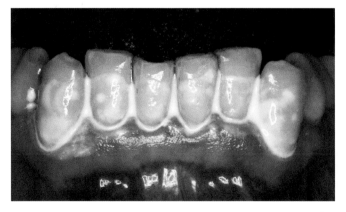
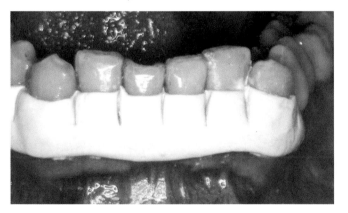

Calxyl is also available in a special syringe equipped with a needle that facilitates the distribution of the product. This is particularly convenient when it is necessary to treat numerous tooth surfaces.

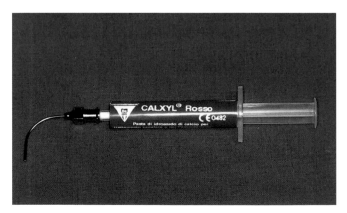
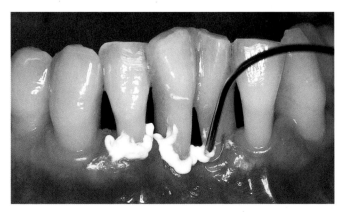

I have obtained excellent results with this method of treatment, and some patients have even ceased to experience problems of hypersensitivity after just one application of calcium hydroxide. In fact, many controlled clinical studies have demonstrated the efficacy of this treatment and its long-lasting effects.[4,6]

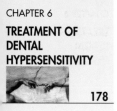
▶ **HOME-CARE APPLICATION**

The patient may use products in the form of gel or toothpaste for self-performed home applications, choosing among those listed below. The efficacy of these products is, however, unpredictable because it is based on the individual response of the patient.

A potassium nitrate gel (Actisens, Byk Gulden, Germany) may be effective for acute symptoms, while toothpaste (Emoform-Actisens, Byk Gulden) is used for maintenance.

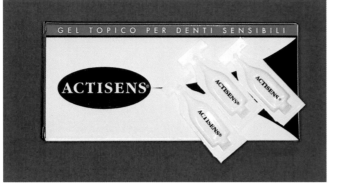

Alternatively, after professional treatment with potassium oxalate performed at the dental office, patients may continue the therapy themselves using the gel toothpaste Protect, which may be applied to the clean tooth surfaces with a finger and then left in place for a few minutes.

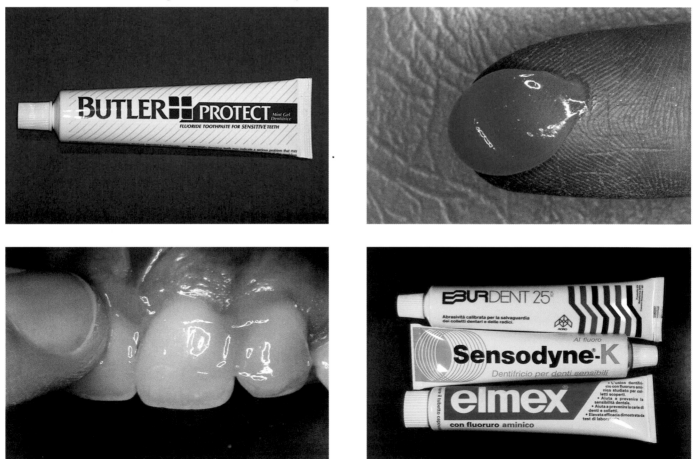

Some other fluoride (Eburdent 25, Betafarma, Italy; Elmex, GABA International, Germany) or strontium chloride (Sensodyne, Block Drug, Jersey City, NJ) toothpastes may also be beneficial for patients.

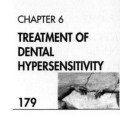
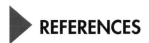 **REFERENCES**

1. Absi EG, Addy M, Adams D. Dentine hypersensitivity. A study of the patency of dentinal tubules in sensitive and non-sensitive cervical dentin. J Clin Periodontol 1987;14:280–284.

2. Addy M, Absi EG, Adams D. Dentine hypersensitivity. The effect in vitro of acids and dietary substances on root-planed and burred dentine. J Clin Periodontol 1987;14:274–279.

3. Brännström M. Sensitivity of dentine. Oral Surg Oral Med Oral Pathol 1966;21:517–526.

4. Green BW, Green ML, McFall WT. Calcium hydroxide and potassium nitrate as desensitizing agents for hypersensitive root surfaces. J Periodontol 1977;48:667–672.

5. Hiatt WH, Johansen E. Root preparation. I. Obturation of dentinal tubules in treatment of root hypersensitivity. J Clin Periodontol 1972;43:373–380.

6. Levin MP, Yearwood LL, Carpenter WN. The desensitizing effect of calcium hydroxide and magnesium hydroxide on hypersensitive dentin. Oral Surg Oral Med Oral Pathol 1973;35:741–746.

7. Lindhe J. Clinical Periodontology and Implant Dentistry, ed 3. Copenhagen: Munksgaard, 1997: chap 9.

8. Orchardson R, Gangarosa LP Sr, Holland GR, et al. Consensus report. Dentine hypersensitivity into the 21st century. Arch Oral Biol 1994;39(suppl):113S–119S.

9. Pashley DH. Dynamics of the pulpo-dentin complex. Crit Rev Oral Biol Med 1996;7:104–133.

**EXPERIENCE
IS THE BEST TEACHER**

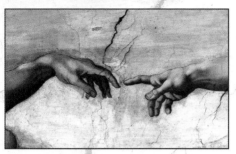

CHAPTER 7

▶ **MAINTENANCE THERAPY
AT TEETH AND IMPLANTS**

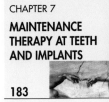
Following cause-related and corrective therapy, maintenance therapy is the phase in which the patient is enrolled in an individually tailored system of periodic recalls aimed at detecting and treating eventual recurrences of the disease and at assessing, and if necessary renewing, the patient's motivation and instruction to improve self-performed plaque control. Maintenance therapy may also be called supportive therapy,[3] because during this phase it is necessary to "support" the patient's efforts to control gingival inflammation.

RESULTS OBTAINED WITH PATIENT PARTICIPATION AND COLLABORATION IN MAINTENANCE THERAPY

The bacteria that cause periodontal disease cannot be completely or definitively eliminated from tooth surfaces. Consequently, professional removal of all microbial deposits in the supragingival and subgingival areas is required at regular intervals. In fact, after the initial procedures of scaling, there will be a recolonization of bacteria that can lead to reinfection and subsequent progression of the disease process in the areas where the patient's self-performed oral hygiene is not sufficiently effective.[30]

Numerous clinical studies have shown that only a program of maintenance therapy aimed at a regular and repeated removal of supragingival and subgingival plaque and at appropriate motivation of the patient can prevent such development over very long periods of time.[4–7,21,23,25,32–35,48,53,58,59] Therefore, regular clinical reevaluations and maintenance care every 3 to 6 months, together with adequate psychologic support, make it possible to maintain the reduced probing depths and gains in clinical attachment obtained after active therapy.[30]

Even after periodontal and prosthetic treatment performed on patients with advanced periodontitis, regular recalls scheduled every 3 to 6 months made it possible to maintain periodontal health for a period of 5 to 8 years.[47] Furthermore, studies have shown that it is possible for almost all patients to maintain for 14 years the results achieved after periodontal treatment.[33] However, it is important to bear in mind that 20% to 25% of patients will exhibit unpredictable reinfection and progression of periodontal lesions in some sites.[30]

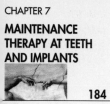
RESULTS OBTAINED WITH PATIENT PARTICIPATION IN MAINTENANCE THERAPY WITHOUT MAINTENANCE OF A SUFFICIENT STANDARD OF ORAL HYGIENE

Although studies have documented the failure of periodontal therapy that is not supported by adequate plaque control,[5,49] results have shown that a maintenance program at regular intervals makes it possible to maintain levels of attachment for many years, even if patients exhibit insufficient oral hygiene.[5,25,44,56] These results indicate that, for a certain period, participation in recalls may compensate for insufficient oral hygiene to a certain extent. This is due to the fact that after professional instrumentation, the quantity and composition of the subgingival flora is modified, and several months may pass before a new deposit forms and triggers subsequent reinfection.[14,36,45] However, individual variations regarding composition, rate of formation of plaque, and defense mechanisms of the host may be observed.[30]

RESULTS OBTAINED WITHOUT PATIENT PARTICIPATION IN MAINTENANCE THERAPY

A study carried out by Nyman et al[48] revealed that patients affected with advanced periodontitis who were treated with surgical techniques but not enrolled in a program of recalls exhibited recurrent periodontitis and further loss of attachment at a much higher rate than that documented for the natural progression of periodontal disease in groups of patients with high disease susceptibility.[37,38]

Furthermore, Axelsson and Lindhe,[4] in a study carried out over a 6-year period, observed the effects produced if patients were not enrolled in an adequate program of maintenance therapy following active therapy. The nonrecalled patients demonstrated signs of recurrent periodontitis at reevaluation 3 and 6 years after active therapy.[30]

Kerr[24] also documented the possibility of recurrent disease in patients who were not enrolled in a program of professional maintenance therapy. Following successful active therapy, patients were referred back to their general dentist, but after 5 years, 45% of the patients exhibited complete reinfection.

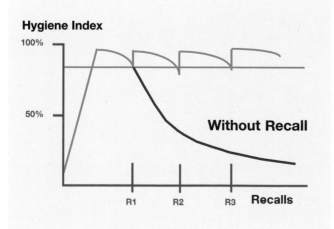

Analogous results have been described for patients who decided not to participate in a professional maintenance program after active periodontal therapy.[10] In fact, the efficacy of motivation and instruction in oral hygiene is short-term for the majority of patients.[18,19] Therefore, without frequent recalls that include reinstruction, patients have a tendency to revert to their old habits relatively quickly.

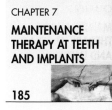

Patients susceptible to periodontitis are at high risk for reinfection and progression of periodontal disease if they do not participate in a well-organized and meticulously performed program of maintenance therapy. All patients treated for periodontitis, and those who may also have undergone prosthetic rehabilitation and implant surgery, require an adequate and individually tailored program of periodic recalls in order to maintain long-term periodontal health after therapy.

▶ PROCEDURES FOR PERIODIC RECALL OF A PATIENT TREATED FOR PERIODONTAL DISEASE

During recall visits, it is advisable to follow a practical plan that may be designed to meet individual needs. In fact, possible omissions may be avoided if the procedures to be performed are organized according to a well-defined plan.

It is advisable to note personal or generic information about patients in their clinical charts so that it is possible to easily reestablish a cordial relationship by showing interest in events mentioned during one of the previous appointments. This type of attention will undoubtedly have a positive effect on the patient's compliance, ie, degree of participation in recalls.

The following procedures are performed during a periodic recall:

• Reevaluation of risk level and periodontal conditions
• Supportive treatment
• Assessment and treatment of recurrence of gingivitis and periodontal disease
• Polishing and treatment of dental hypersensitivity

▷ REEVALUATION OF RISK LEVEL AND PERIODONTAL CONDITIONS

During the initial periodontal examination, the entity of the disease is determined by assessing the loss of clinical attachment, the depth of the periodontal pockets, and the degree of inflammation. The first recall is scheduled 3 months after the conclusion of active periodontal treatment, and during this visit the clinical parameters are carefully reevaluated and compared to the initial data recorded in the patient's clinical chart. Subsequently, during each recall the dentist and the hygienist must gather all clinical data that may be an early indication of a new onset or recurrence of the periodontal disease in a previously treated site. The clinical parameters gathered at successive reevaluations must always be compared with the data registered during the previous recall.

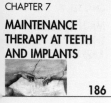
Preferably, the same hygienist should follow the patient in the course of both active and maintenance therapy; it is, however, the dentist who is responsible for the treatment and who must personally examine the patient during the first reevaluation, at regular intervals during maintenance therapy, and whenever the hygienist observes problems that require a consultation. It is essential for the dentist to monitor not only the state of health of the hard and soft tissue, but also the patient's degree of oral hygiene so that the important effect of this parameter on oral health can be emphasized. If the patient's case history indicates susceptibility to periodontitis, it is important to determine the risk of reinfection and/or progression of the disease, evaluating at the subject, tooth, and site levels.[30]

The factors to be evaluated at the subject level are:

- Systemic conditions, updating all clinical data regarding their general health status, and any medicines that they may be consuming
- Lifestyle factors that may be relevant, such as stress and smoking; heavy smokers are considered at high risk for reinfection[13]
- Degree of participation in periodic recalls (compliance)

After registering the above-mentioned data in the patient's clinical chart, the following clinical examinations should be performed at the tooth and site levels[30]:

- Gingival Bleeding Index (GBI)
- Plaque Index (PI)
- Probing depth with scoring of pockets and bleeding on probing (BOP)
- Gingival recessions
- Furcation involvement
- Tooth mobility
- Plaque-retention factors
- Gingival lesions
- Caries and radiographic examinations

Multilevel risk analysis makes it possible to reevaluate simultaneously the level of risk for reinfection and/or progression of the disease and the patient's status of dental health.

The above-mentioned examination is performed according to the methods of execution and interpretation described in Chapter 1. The results obtained are never absolute, but must always be evaluated in relation to the data registered at previous appointments.

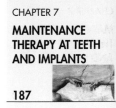
GINGIVAL BLEEDING INDEX[2]

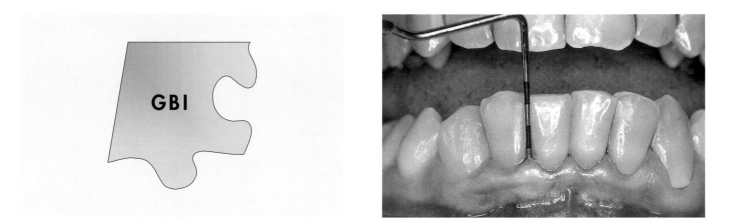

The Gingival Bleeding Index exactly expresses the extent of gingivitis and aims at reevaluating the patient's level of collaboration. Patients with a low index may be considered at low risk for reinfection.[26]

PLAQUE INDEX[52]

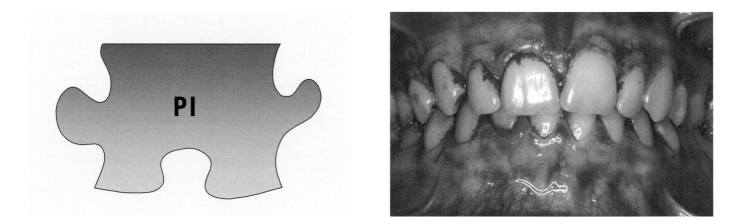

This index exactly expresses patients' manual ability to clean their teeth. Bacterial plaque causes inflammation that may be more or less evident in relation to the host response of the patient. It is important to understand that the plaque index must always be evaluated in relation to the host response of the patient, which means that it must be compared to the Gingival Bleeding Index. In fact, monitoring may reveal absence of plaque, but presence of bleeding along the gingival margin; this indicates that the patient removed the plaque just a short while before the recall so there was not enough time for the inflammation to subside. Therefore, the most reliable clinical parameter in determining the patient's level of cooperation and possible risk of reinfection is the Gingival Bleeding Index.

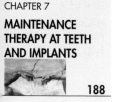
PROBING DEPTH WITH SCORING OF POCKETS AND BLEEDING ON PROBING

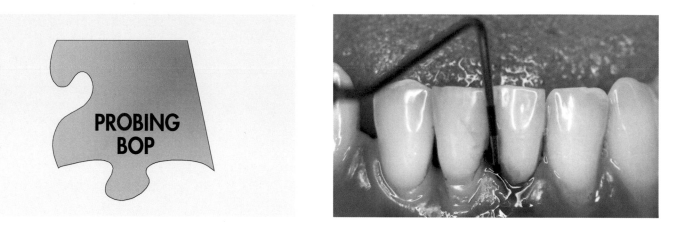

Clinical probing is the most commonly used procedure to evaluate the condition of the periodontal tissues. The presence of numerous deep pockets that increase in depth during maintenance therapy is indicative of high risk for disease progression.[8,16]

It is very important to detect the sites that bleed upon deep probing. It is necessary to apply a light pressure of 25 g during probing. This is the most reliable standard force used to detect sites that bleed.[29] If a force superior to 25 g were applied, bleeding might be caused by trauma and not by the presence of infection in the site.

Absence of bleeding on probing is indicative of periodontal stability.[26,27] On the other hand, bleeding on probing indicates presence of gingival inflammation and implies that there are deposits of subgingival plaque and calculus. There seems to be a higher risk for progression of periodontitis in sites that bleed, especially when this sign is repeatedly present in successive reevaluations.[16,27]

GINGIVAL RECESSIONS

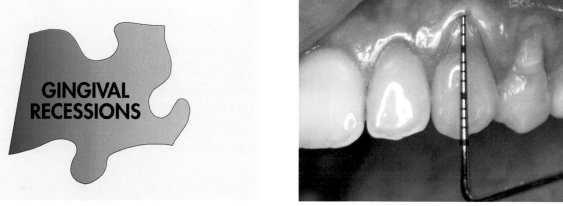

Gingival recessions are monitored with the graduated probe, taking the measurement from the cementoenamel junction to the bottom of the pocket or sulcus to verify if there has been further loss of clinical attachment.

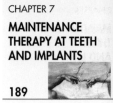

FURCATION INVOLVEMENT

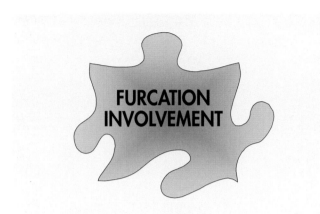

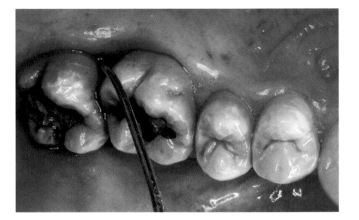

Furcation involvement must be monitored or detected in a careful examination of the periodontal status of multirooted teeth. Analyses have established that multirooted teeth with furcation involvement seem to be at high risk for disease progression during the maintenance phase.[22,41] In fact, when treatment outcomes are evaluated on the basis of bleeding frequency, probing depth reductions, and levels of attachment, there are noticeable differences between the results obtained in furcation sites and those obtained in single-rooted sites and flat molar surfaces.[39,46,55] Nevertheless, studies have shown that if a series of well-organized recalls is scheduled for the patient, the prognosis may be considered quite good.

TOOTH MOBILITY

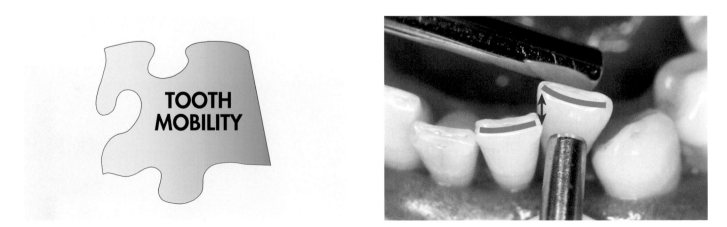

Tooth mobility must also be evaluated. Increased mobility may be a sign that periodontal damage is progressing; in this case, the hygienist's task is to advise the dentist.

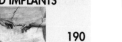
PLAQUE RETENTION FACTORS

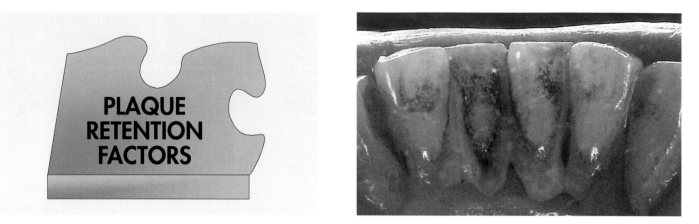

Retentive factors, such as calculus and overhanging restorations, facilitate accumulations of plaque. Presence of calculus indicates poor oral hygiene and insufficient collaboration on the part of the patient.

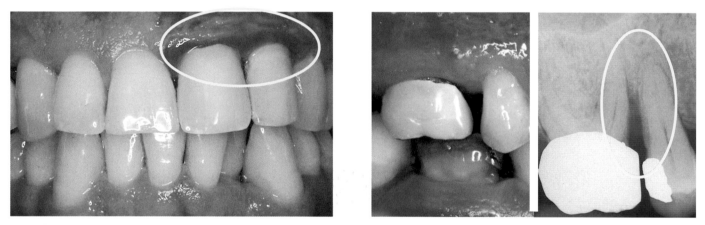

Overhanging restorations and ill-fitting crown margins represent an area for plaque retention and provide more favorable conditions for the establishment of gram-negative anaerobic microbiota,[28] which increases the risk for periodontal destruction.

GINGIVAL LESIONS

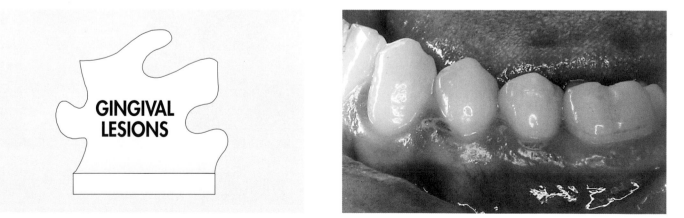

The presence of trauma caused by excessively vigorous or incorrect toothbrushing, or other lesions that may be the result of improper oral hygiene practices, must be monitored; if such signs are detected, the patient must be corrected and reinstructed.

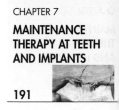
CARIES AND RADIOGRAPHIC EXAMINATIONS

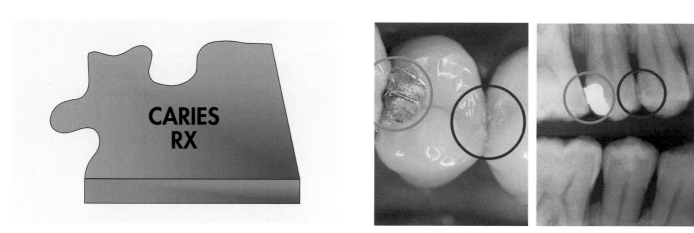

Caries and other pathologic factors should be detected to evaluate the variations in the patient's dental status that occur in the course of time.

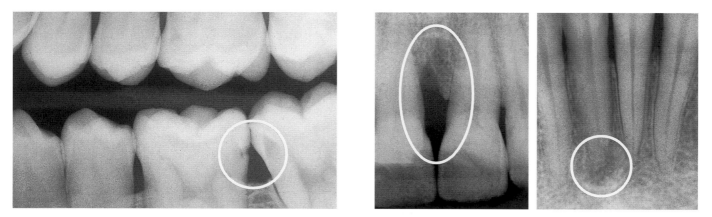

Radiographic surveys should be carried out every 2 to 4 years if no complications arise. These examinations will supply important information regarding caries, possible progression of periodontal disease, and the presence of any apical lesions.

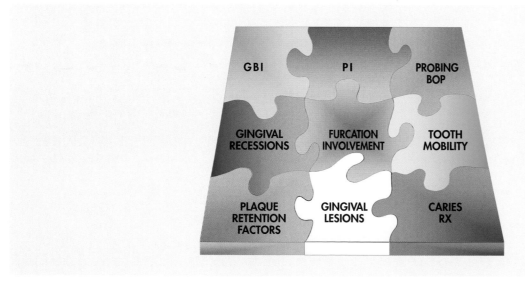

At this point, all clinical data have been gathered, and the information is recorded in the patient's periodontal chart. A new periodontal chart is compiled at each recall.

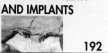
Software by ARDEC, distributed by Arminium Odontologica srl, Italy, www.ardec.it.

Recall of Dental Hygiene

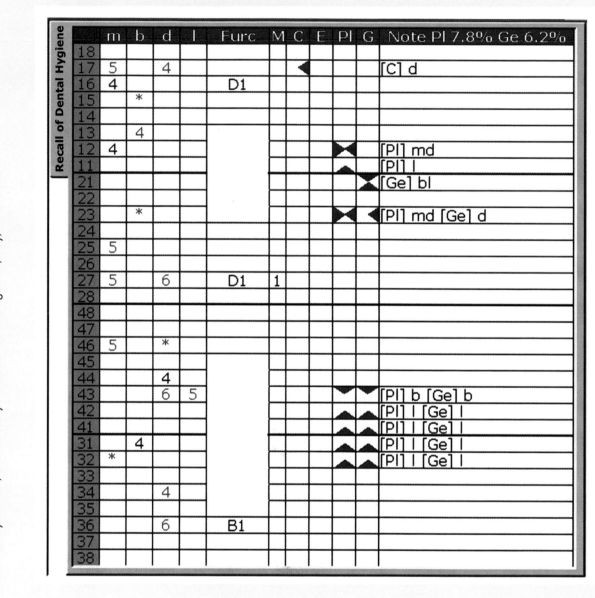

	m	b	d	l	Furc	M	C	E	Pl	G	Note Pl 7.8% Ge 6.2%
18											
17	5		4				◀				[C] d
16	4				D1						
15		*									
14											
13		4									
12	4								✕		[Pl] md
11									▲		[Pl] l
21									✕		[Ge] bl
22											
23		*							✕	◀	[Pl] md [Ge] d
24											
25	5										
26											
27	5		6		D1	1					
28											
48											
47											
46	5		*								
45											
44			4								
43			6	5					▼	▼	[Pl] b [Ge] b
42									▲	▲	[Pl] l [Ge] l
41									▲	▲	[Pl] l [Ge] l
31			4						▲	▲	[Pl] l [Ge] l
32	*								▲	▲	[Pl] l [Ge] l
33											
34			4								
35											
36			6		B1						
37											
38											

An evaluation of risk at the subject, tooth, and site levels and the reevaluation of the patient's periodontal conditions determine the overall risk profile and the extent and frequency of the maintenance therapy required.

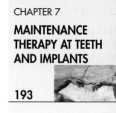
▷ SUPPORTIVE TREATMENT

REINFORCEMENT OF MOTIVATION

Patients want and need to be informed about their dental health and the results of their home-care efforts. If the hygienist does not satisfy this need, patients may get the impression that the hygienist has lost interest in their problems, and this may have a negative effect on motivation and compliance with recalls.

Those patients who make a great effort to perform the suggested home-care procedures and who have undergone long treatments at the dental office want particular attention and encouragement. The patient should be informed about the clinical results gathered during the recall visit. The hygienist should point out in particular the sites that bleed on probing and the number of pockets > 4 mm, reminding the patient of the reasons for which these clinical signs still persist. Patients will be satisfied if the scores are low, but will be discouraged if they are high and the presence of periodontal pockets is detected. Patients who have neglected to perform adequate hygiene practices need to be further motivated; while carrying out this task, the hygienist should make an effort to understand the reasons for their lack of collaboration.

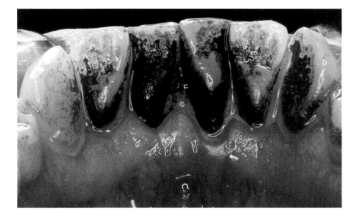

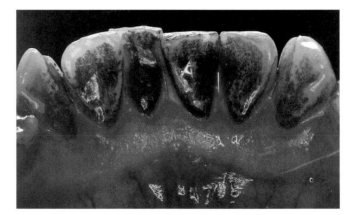

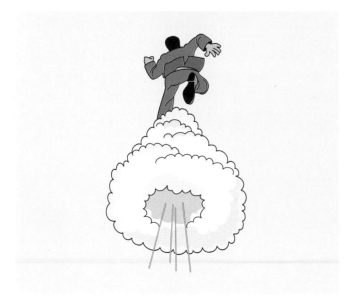

Further motivation may be tiresome and boring for the hygienist, and if this repetition is based on criticism, patients may be offended. This type of motivation is not usually effective and may discourage patients from complying with further recalls. Motivation must be constructive so that patients are aware that the hygienist is still interested in their periodontal and dental health. The same strategies used during the patient's first appointment are also necessary when further motivation is required, and the mutual trust that has been established between patient and hygienist will facilitate a spontaneous and friendly dialogue.

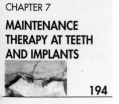
In the majority of cases, an adequate approach enables the hygienist to obtain the desired results. Many patients neglect proper care of their oral cavities before they become aware of their problem, but after motivation and adequate instruction, they are able to maintain a good level of oral hygiene.

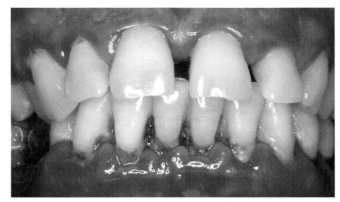
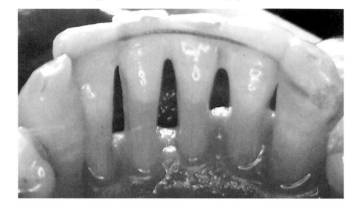

Some patients are so motivated that they are able to maintain perfect dental health and therefore do not need particularly extensive treatment during recalls.

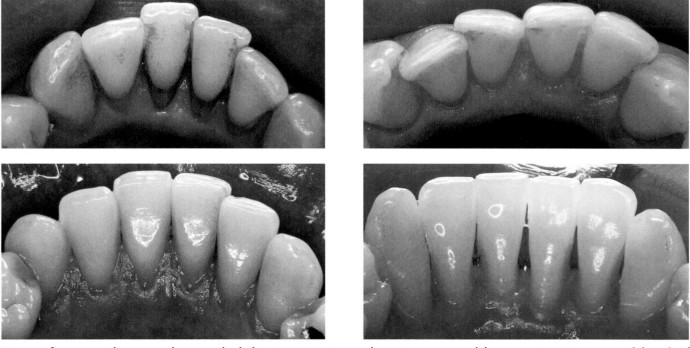

Even after complex prosthetic rehabilitation, motivated patients are able to maintain a good level of hygiene.

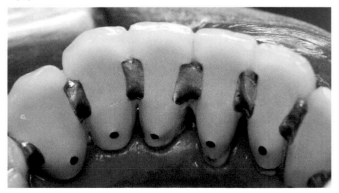
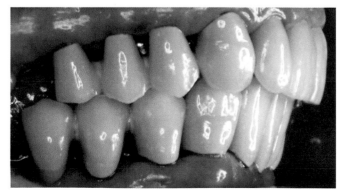

REINSTRUCTION IN PLAQUE CONTROL

The data gathered in the patient's chart may indicate that the patient requires further instruction aimed at improving self-performed plaque control in sites that present signs of inflammation. Several important aspects must be considered in order to make this reinstruction more effective and helpful.

In some cases, the patient may lack the manual dexterity required to carry out the previously recommended hygiene practices. In other cases, the home-care program may not have been performed regularly. Sometimes, particular situations concerning the patient's private life may have had a negative influence on collaboration. In any case, encouragement from the hygienist is always advisable in the attempt to obtain the patient's collaboration.

After active periodontal therapy, the morphology of the patient's gingivae may have changed, making it necessary to substitute some of the oral hygiene instruments that were previously recommended and to introduce new ones. These variations are frequent in the interproximal areas, where the spaces between teeth become wider after active therapy.

The placement of new prosthetic devices may render the use of adjunctive instruments necessary. Furthermore, the neck area of treated teeth may be hypersensitive, making it difficult for the patient to perform the proper oral hygiene practices. Consequently, treatment for dental hypersensitivity is required to reduce or eliminate the patient's discomfort and enable the level of plaque control to be improved. The patient must also be corrected if signs of trauma caused by incorrect hygiene practices are visible.

▷ ASSESSMENT AND TREATMENT OF RECURRENCE OF GINGIVITIS AND PERIODONTAL DISEASE

If the outcome of treatment was positive but the patient later presents symptoms of the disease again, this must be considered a sign of reinfection, which is termed "recurrence." Many different factors may cause this reinfection.

The patient may have had problems in maintaining a good level of oral hygiene, or may have failed to comply regularly with the recommended program of periodic recalls. In either case, the hygienist must understand the reasons for the patient's lack of collaboration. Alternatively, the patient may have complied with recalls regularly but may not have received adequate periodontal treatment; in fact, if the examination and reevaluation of the periodontal conditions were not appropriate and the subsequent treatment was consequently inadequate, recurrence is more likely to occur.

Some important assessments must be made if recurrence is exhibited. It is necessary to:

• Distinguish between generalized or local reinfection
• Analyze factors that may have caused the reinfection
• Choose, in collaboration with the dentist, the most suitable treatment for the reinfected sites

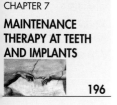
GENERALIZED REINFECTION

Signs of generalized gingivitis that reappear at a regular recall do not necessarily indicate that there is a recurrence of periodontal disease; this situation may be the result of the patient's momentary negligence in performing adequate hygiene procedures. After further motivation, any deposits of plaque and calculus are removed with the sickle and the sonic unit. The patient will then be recalled after 3 months.

However, the presence of extensive bleeding and periodontal pockets > 4 mm indicate a recurrence of periodontitis. This may be due to insufficient maintenance therapy and poor motivation on the part of the patient, who therefore requires more frequent periodic recalls. In fact, it is important to keep patients previously treated for advanced periodontal disease under very strict observation.[54,59] As mentioned previously, due consideration must always be given to patients' level of risk, which is in part determined by systemic conditions and lifestyle factors that may render them particularly susceptible to the disease.

After further motivation, accumulations of plaque and calculus are removed utilizing curettes, a sickle, and an ultrasonic or sonic unit. Instrumentation under local anesthesia is recommended for pockets > 5 mm, and use of adjunctive therapy such as antibiotics may be useful.[30] The dentist will determine the most adequate treatment and indicate whether systemic or local administration is more appropriate.

Furthermore, root planing should be performed very carefully to protect the hard tissues. In fact, the intentional removal of "altered cementum" is not justified during maintenance therapy,[43,50,51] just as it is not justified during the active phase of therapy. Only those sites that exhibit signs of inflammation, ie, all sites and all periodontal pockets that bleed on probing, have to be retreated with subgingival instrumentation. Repeated instrumentation of healthy sites would inevitably cause continuous loss of probing attachment.[34] Therefore, these nonbleeding sites should only be polished at the end of the appointment.

Caries may also be monitored during treatment. Interproximal caries may often be detected during instrumentation with curettes. The dentist will decide if urgent treatment is required.

If the recurrence of periodontal disease is at an initial stage, the patient's next recall should be scheduled after 3 months. During this visit, the hygienist will monitor the efficacy of the patient's daily oral hygiene practices and the results of the further treatment that was performed.

If, instead, the recurrence is advanced, it is advisable to recall the patient after about 1 month in order to monitor the level of cooperation and the results of the further periodontal treatment. The results achieved will help the dentist to determine the further therapy required. Surgical treatment will only be scheduled if patients are able to maintain a good level of oral hygiene; otherwise, their treatment will be limited to frequently planned recalls with the hygienist.

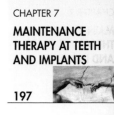
LOCAL REINFECTION

Local recurrence of periodontal disease is usually caused by inadequate plaque control in a certain area. The patient's oral hygiene practices may have been inadequate in sites where retention factors such as calculus, overhanging restorations, and ecologic niches are present, or in areas that are inaccessible, such as furcations. These sites require thorough instrumentation that is often performed under local anesthesia. Sometimes, the local application of antibiotics is useful as an adjunct, as in the case presented below.

During a regular recall, the patient, previously treated for periodontitis gravis, exhibited reinfection in the mesiobuccal site of tooth 37, with clinical probing of 10 mm also documented by the radiographic examination that revealed a mesial angular defect at tooth 37.

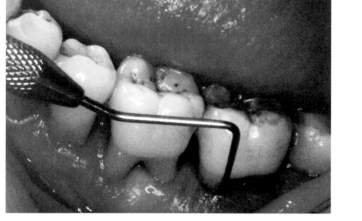

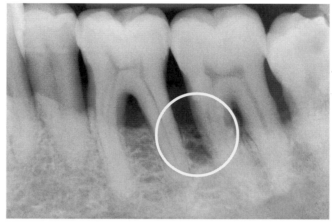

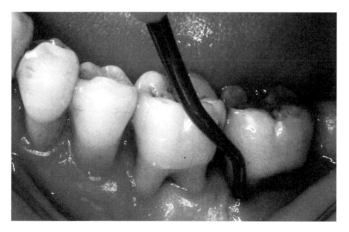

The dentist planned the repetition of scaling procedures under local anesthesia and also introduced local application of a gel containing 25% metronidazole (Elyzol, Dumex-Alpharma, Denmark). I retreated the site following the dentist's indications, and at the subsequent recall after 3 months, the clinical probing depth was reduced to 3 mm. The radiographic examination 6 months after treatment confirmed the successful outcome of the treatment, revealing bone apposition and closure of the angular defect.

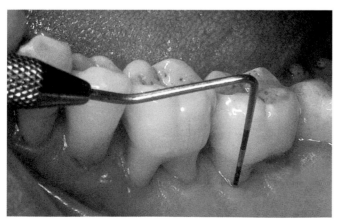

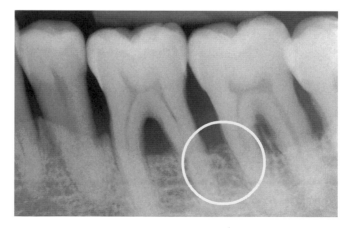

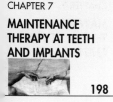
In other cases, the dentist may decide that cleaning with surgical access is required; this surgical treatment is necessary when not only bleeding on probing but also further loss of attachment in the same site are exhibited at various consecutive recalls. However, if recurrent infection is the result of inadequate oral hygiene, the surgical procedure must be postponed until the patient's plaque control has reached acceptable levels.

It is important to bear in mind that the sites that do not respond to therapy and that evidence further loss of clinical attachment may represent cases in which bacteria remained inside the dentin[1] and then returned outside, through the dentinal tubules, to reinfect the periodontal tissue. In these cases, scaling is performed, and topical or systemic antibiotic therapy may be introduced to improve the effect of the treatment.

▷ POLISHING AND TREATMENT OF DENTAL HYPERSENSITIVITY

Final polishing with polishing paste is recommended to remove all residual soft deposits and stains; this procedure also gives the patient a pleasant sensation of freshness in the oral cavity. If certain areas exhibit dental hypersensitivity, products that have the potential to close the dentinal tubules (eg, potassium oxalate, sodium fluoride, calcium hydroxide) should be chosen and applied. Instructions for the use of these products are supplied in Chapter 6.

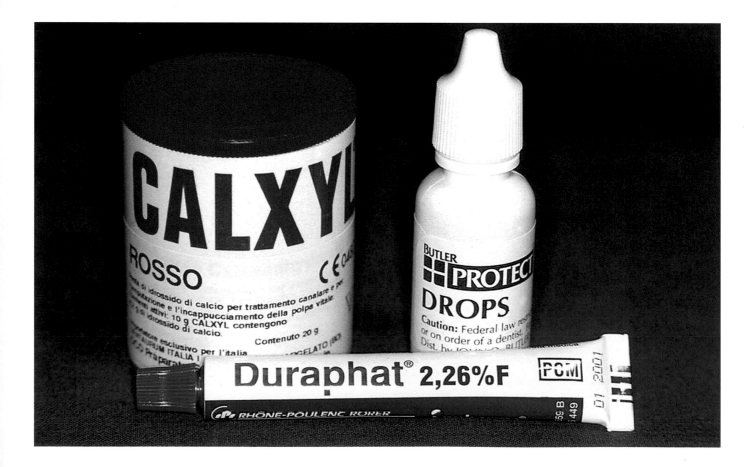

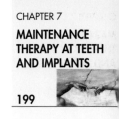

MAINTENANCE THERAPY AT IMPLANTS

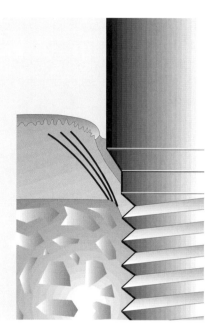

An essential element for a long-term prognosis of implant-supported restorations is the health of peri-implant tissues.[30] Appropriate and regular oral hygiene practices are essential because plaque is substantially similar at implant sites and periodontal sites. The onset and the progression of a peri-implant infection has the same clinical, histologic, and microbiologic evolution as that of a periodontal lesion,[11,12,20,31] but the extent of tissue breakdown is more evident around implants than it is around teeth.[31] Therefore, the bacterial plaque situated around the peri-implant mucosa may also cause inflammation, which may lead to failure of the therapy and loss of the implant.[57]

Consequently, it is very important that patients with implants comply with recalls scheduled by the dentist and hygienist to maintain the outcome of the treatment performed. Following active treatment, the first year of maintenance therapy requires one recall every 3 to 4 months; the frequency of subsequent recalls will be scheduled according to each patient's ability to maintain a good level of plaque control. However, I recommend at least two annual recalls so that the hygienist can clean the abutments meticulously. One annual checkup by the dentist is also advisable to monitor occlusion and perform radiographic examinations if necessary.

PROCEDURES FOR PERIODIC RECALL OF A PATIENT WITH IMPLANTS

The following procedures are performed during the periodic recall:

- Examination and reevaluation of the peri-implant mucosa and plaque control
- Supportive treatment
- Treatment of possible mucositis
- Polishing of implants and prostheses

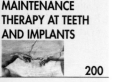
▷ **EXAMINATION AND REEVALUATION OF THE PERI-IMPLANT MUCOSA AND PLAQUE CONTROL**

At each recall, it is necessary to reevaluate the condition of the tissue of the peri-implant mucosa by running a plastic probe along the margin of the mucosa and scoring the presence or absence of bleeding. This examination may be undertaken around all abutments, no matter which type of prosthetic device has been placed. A plastic probe is utilized to avoid damaging the titanium surfaces whether in the presence of a complete-arch prosthesis, a partial prosthesis,

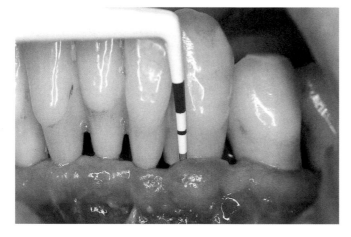
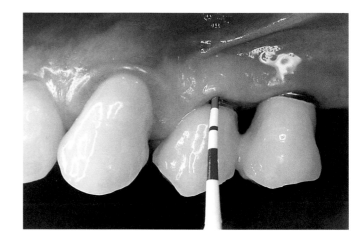

a Toronto structure, a double structure, or an overdenture.

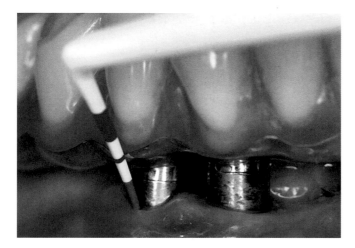
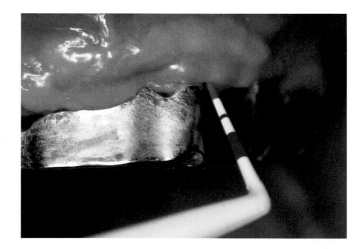

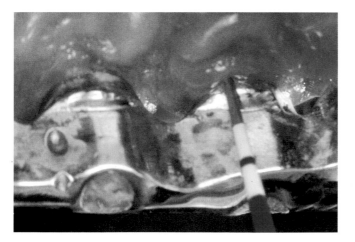
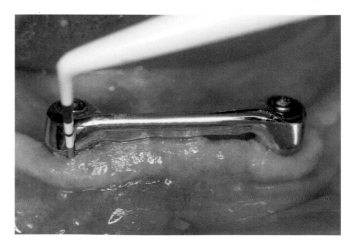

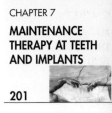
This method can be used to determine the level of cooperation of patients with implants, and it is similar to the method used to determine the same factor in periodontally compromised patients. It is also necessary to evaluate:

- Presence or absence of plaque and calculus
- Presence or absence of suppuration
- Clinical mobility of the implant
- Resorption of the alveolar bone

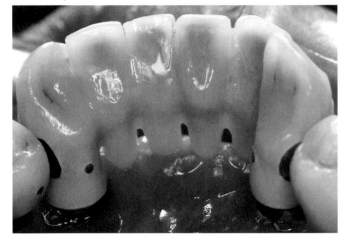

The hygienist's task is to maintain the peri-implant mucosa in a healthy condition, with no signs of inflammation. Therefore, bleeding along the margin of the mucosa and plaque accumulation must be carefully monitored.

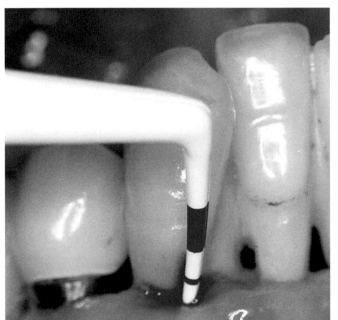

If obvious signs of change, such as profuse bleeding, edema, erythema, fistulae, or mobility, are visible, the hygienist must advise the dentist, who will perform peri-implant clinical probing, compare it to the radiographic examination, and act accordingly to resolve the inflammation.

▷ **SUPPORTIVE TREATMENT**

If required, the patient will have to be further motivated, and the reasons the patient was not able to maintain a good level of plaque control around the implants must be determined. Then, the motivation must be reinforced in relation to the cause of the negligence (see the previous section on supportive treatment, pp 193 to 195).

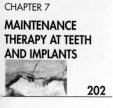
▷ TREATMENT OF POSSIBLE MUCOSITIS

When performing maintenance therapy on implants, the task of the hygienist is limited to treating mucositis, ie, the inflammatory reaction of the soft tissues that surround the implant.[30] The treatment of peri-implantitis, ie, the process of infection that causes the loss of bone around the implant,[30] is the task of the dentist alone.

The removal of plaque and calculus from the area surrounding the abutments requires appropriate procedures in order to preserve the original smoothness of the titanium for as long as possible. Titanium can be easily scratched, creating a rough surface that therefore facilitates plaque retention.

Spongy floss or gauze floss can be used to remove plaque from abutments because these types of floss can easily surround the abutments.

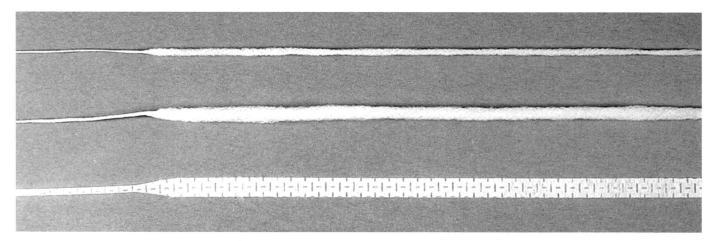

The two extremities of the floss are crossed like a necktie, then slid around the implant.

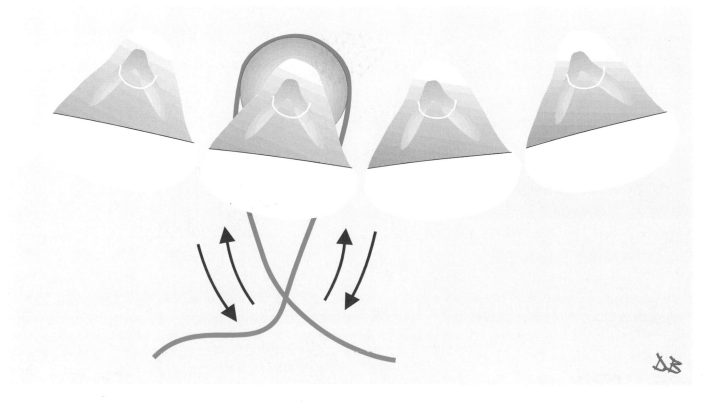

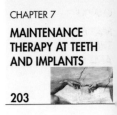

The choice of floss depends on the width of the space between the peri-implant mucosa and the prosthesis.

Spongy floss (Super-floss, Oral-B, Boston, MA) is used when the space is narrow.

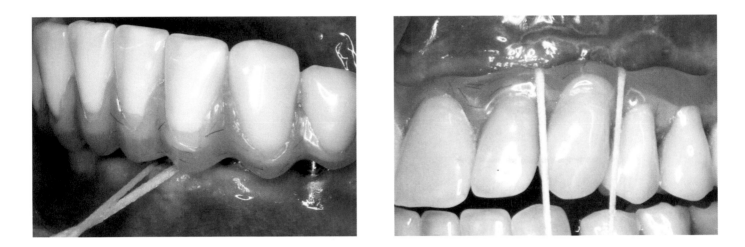

This technique is used on each implant, winding the floss around the abutment both from the buccal side and from the lingual side.

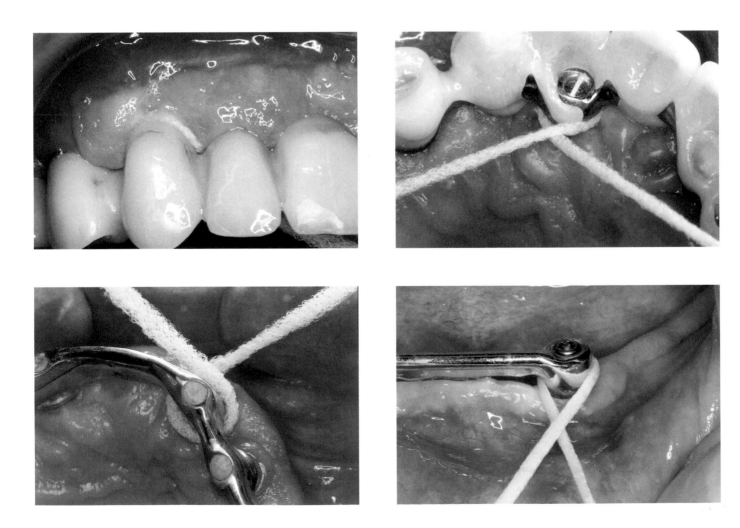

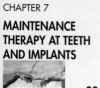
If the procedures are very difficult, small tweezers or a threader can be used to facilitate the passage of the Super-floss.

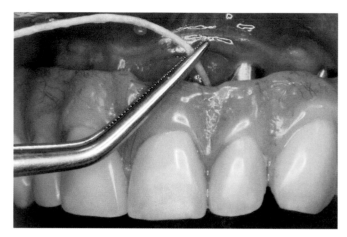

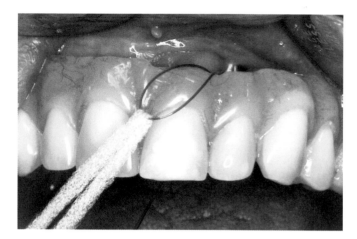

If the space is wide enough, a more spongy floss (Thornton International, Norwalk, CT) may be used.

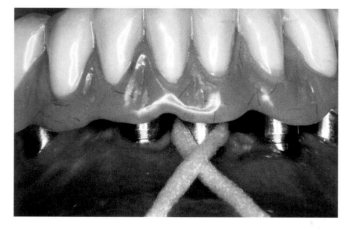

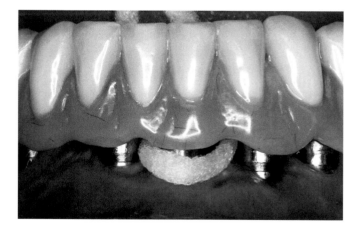

Or, if the space is very wide, the use of gauze floss (G-Floss, Hygiene Systems, West Palm Beach, FL) is recommended.

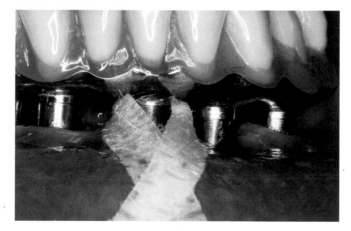

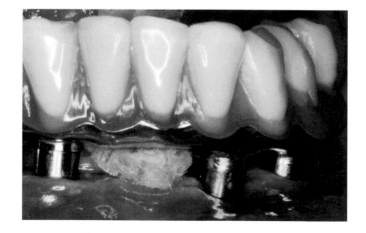

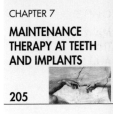
Steel curettes and ultrasonic devices cannot be used to remove any deposits of calculus that may have formed on the abutments, since these instruments would scratch the surface of the titanium.[40] Curettes in various forms have been devised expressly for this purpose; they remove the calculus but do not damage the surface of the implants. These instruments may be made of carbon fibers (Hawe Neos Dental, Switzerland), acetate (Nobel Biocare, Sweden), gold (Implant Innovations Inc, Palm Beach Gardens, FL), or titanium (Deppeler, Switzerland). If the curette selected has the same design as a universal curette, it is possible to clean all areas of the oral cavity with adequate access.

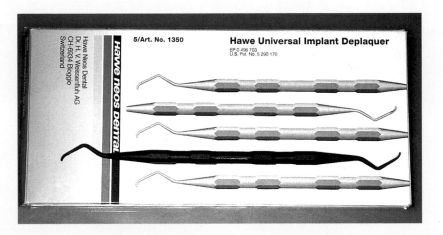

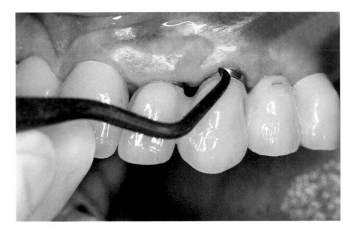

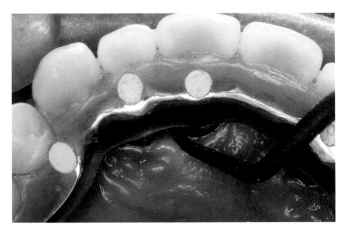

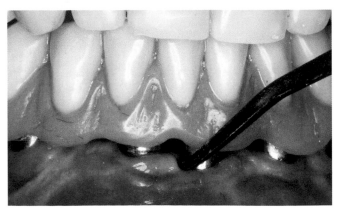

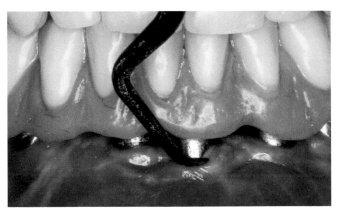

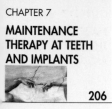
If a substantial quantity of calculus has formed around the implant, scaling can be performed effectively with a mechanical sonic vibration instrument (SONICflex, KaVo, Germany) that is equipped with a metal point covered with a plastic single-use insert (Densonic Softip, Dentstply, York, PA).

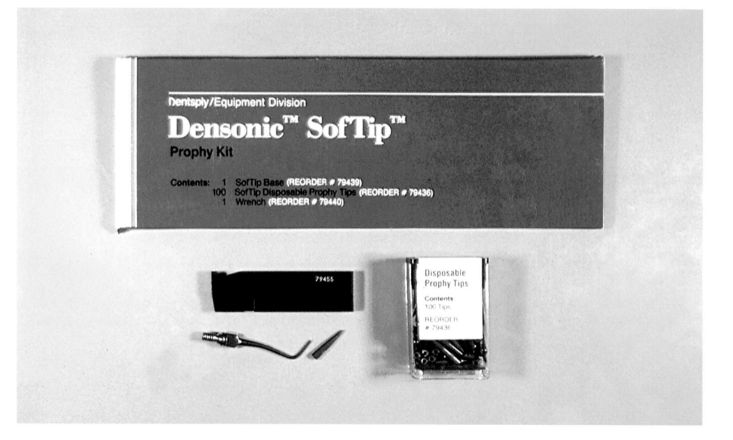

This instrument is very effective in the removal of plaque and calculus and does not alter the surfaces of titanium implants.[40]

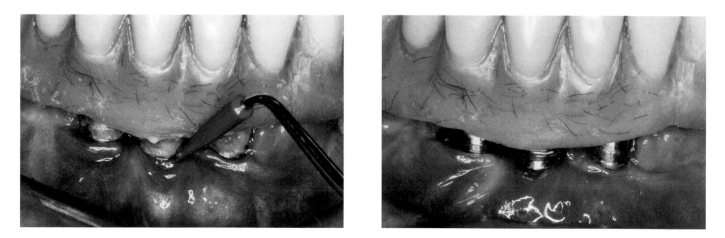

▷ POLISHING OF IMPLANTS AND PROSTHESES

Special brushes or rubber cups inserted in a handpiece are used to polish implants. These instruments make it easier to pass between abutments, and they are used with polishing paste with a low degree of abrasiveness (eg, RDA 8.9).

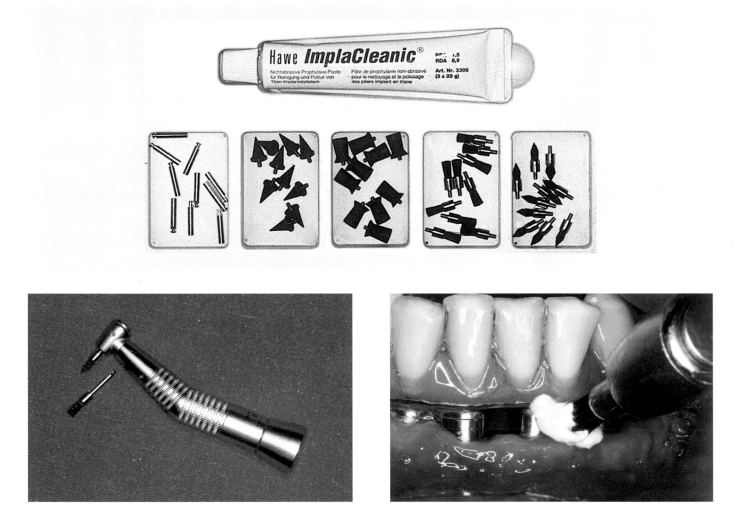

When the crown of an implant prosthesis fits perfectly with the margin of the mucosa, the rubber cup is used with the same technique utilized on natural elements.

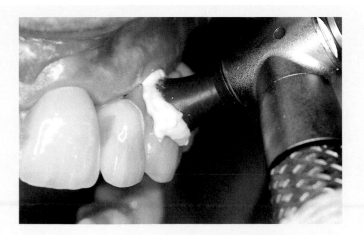

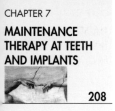
▶ HOW TO ORGANIZE AN EFFICIENT HYGIENE SERVICE

Recalls during maintenance therapy should be scheduled on the basis of the patient's susceptibility to periodontal disease, which is determined by the risk at the subject level and the careful reevaluation of the clinical parameters scored at each recall.

Initially, patients with advanced periodontitis may require recalls every 3 to 4 months. Subsequently, the lapse of time between these recalls may be shortened or lengthened according to the results obtained. It is very important to carefully evaluate the patient's ability to maintain an adequate standard of oral hygiene and the number of sites that still exhibit bleeding on probing. Patients with inadequate plaque control and/or a high percentage of bleeding sites should be recalled more frequently than patients who exhibit excellent plaque control and healthy gingival tissue.

An efficient hygiene service must be organized to maintain a high percentage of patient compliance. This service must satisfy the requirements of all patients, and it must be timely and precise. Good software that can program periodic recalls is extremely helpful in this sense. Patients may be advised by mail or by telephone that they are due for a recall.

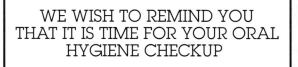

WE WISH TO REMIND YOU
THAT IT IS TIME FOR YOUR ORAL
HYGIENE CHECKUP

We advise you to make an
appointment as soon as possible.

BEST REGARDS

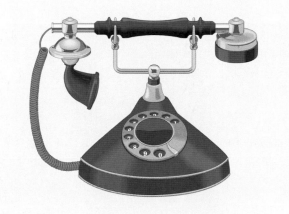

I personally use the first method, and I usually send a simple note reminding the patient to make an appointment. I prefer to leave patients free to decide if they want to comply with the recall. Patients must not feel that they are under obligation; however, their level of participation will depend on the efficacy of the motivation provided by the hygienist during active therapy.

The telephone message implies more involvement on the part of patients, who may, however, accept the suggestion to schedule an appointment only because they are ashamed to refuse; the goal is not to "force" them to comply with recalls!

This problem of recalling the patients does not exist if the patients themselves promptly ask to schedule their next appointment. This usually happens when they are extremely motivated and consider recalls a permanent commitment necessary to maintain their oral health.

In order to help patients to remember their appointments, it is better to phone them a few days in advance to remind them about the date of their periodic recall. Sometimes, the patients themselves request this reminder.

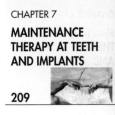

A readily available supply of all instruments and products that are necessary for self-performed oral hygiene is an additional service that must be offered to satisfy patients' requirements.

▶ PATIENT COMPLIANCE WITH MAINTENANCE PROGRAMS

Studies have widely documented that patients who have undergone periodontal therapy and who comply with regular recalls have a better prognosis than those who do not collaborate.[4,10,24,42] Those who exhibit "irregular" compliance, or do not follow a program of maintenance therapy, may have a high level of risk for the progression of periodontal disease. Unfortunately, numerous clinical studies[15,17,42,61] have shown that only a minority of periodontal patients comply with the recommended program of maintenance therapy. These studies supply a good example of the difference that exists between our expectations and clinical reality. Despite the hygienist's efforts to encourage compliance, many patients may not follow the necessary program of periodic recalls.

There are many reasons for this noncompliance,[60] and they may derive from any of the following facts:

- Patients do not receive adequate information about their disease.
- Patients do not understand the hygienist's message.
- Patients do not feel that the disease is particularly threatening to their oral health.
- Patients' anxiety is not adequately soothed, and they continue to fear treatment.

All of these factors may derive from an inadequate approach during active therapy. However, regardless of therapeutic shortcomings, patients also lacked the motivation necessary to induce them to follow the program of periodontal therapy. The information given to patients must always be supported by their own desire to modify their incorrect habits.

Another important aspect that sometimes determines noncompliance may be patients' financial situations, which could impede them from complying with their periodic recalls, even though they may be motivated.[60] Furthermore, a study conducted by Becker et al[9] revealed that patients who did not participate in a program of maintenance therapy after active periodontal treatment were those who were previously less successful in life, less tolerant, more aggressive, and led more stressful lives with unstable interpersonal relationships.

Naturally, each hygienist really wants to do everything possible to help patients affected with periodontal disease; however, once the active phase of treatment has been completed, the long-term prognosis essentially depends on the patient's behavior and collaboration. The efficacy of the message and the enthusiasm that the hygienist conveys cannot guarantee infallible results, but in many cases, they can be decisive in stimulating patients to collaborate to preserve their teeth.

▶ **TABLES OF REFERENCE**

The following table presents the procedures that should be performed during the periodic recall of a patient affected with periodontal disease.

REEVALUATION OF LEVEL OF RISK AND PERIODONTAL CONDITIONS

AT SUBJECT LEVEL

- Assessment of patients' general health status, consumption of medicines, stress, smoking, and compliance

AT TOOTH AND SITE LEVEL

- Gingival Bleeding Index
- Plaque Index
- Probing depth with scoring of pockets and bleeding on probing
- Gingival recessions
- Furcation involvement
- Tooth mobility
- Plaque-retention factors
- Gingival lesions
- Caries and radiographic examinations (if necessary)

COMPARE THE CLINICAL DATA OBTAINED AT EACH RECALL TO THE PARAMETERS REGISTERED AT THE PREVIOUS VISIT

ASSESSMENT OF THE COLLABORATION AND SUPPORTIVE TREATMENT REQUIRED

- Analyze the reasons for lack of collaboration if the patient exhibits insufficient oral hygiene
- Reinforce motivation
- Repeat instructions in plaque control
- Substitute, if necessary, some of the instruments for home care in cases where the morphology of the gingiva has changed
- Introduce new instruments if necessary

ASSESSMENT AND TREATMENT OF RECURRENT GINGIVITIS AND PERIODONTAL DISEASE

- Distinguish between generalized and local recurrence
- Analyze the possible causes of reinfection
- Perform the proper treatment indicated by the dentist

POLISHING OF THE DENTAL SURFACES

- Remove any residual deposits and stains
- Choose and apply specific products for symptoms of dental hypersensitivity that may be exhibited in certain areas of the oral cavity

SCHEDULING OF THE NEXT RECALL

HEALTHY PERIODONTIUM
GINGIVITIS
PERIODONTITIS LEVIS
PERIODONTITIS GRAVIS

- Recall after 6 months
- Recall after 3 months
- Recall after 3 months
- Recall after 1 month

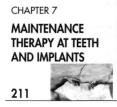

The following table presents the procedures that should be performed during the periodic recall of a patient who has undergone implant surgery.

EXAMINATION AND REEVALUATION OF THE PERI-IMPLANT MUCOSA AND PLAQUE CONTROL

- Condition of the tissue of the peri-implant mucosa
- Presence or absence of plaque and/or calculus
- Presence or absence of suppuration
- Clinical mobility of the implant
- Resorption of the alveolar bone

COMPARE THE DATA OBTAINED AT EACH RECALL TO THE PARAMETERS REGISTERED AT THE PREVIOUS VISIT

ASSESSMENT OF THE COLLABORATION AND SUPPORTIVE TREATMENT REQUIRED

- Analyze the reasons for lack of collaboration if the patient exhibits insufficient oral hygiene
- Reinforce motivation
- Repeat instructions in plaque control
- Substitute, if necessary, some of the instruments for home care in cases where the morphology of the gingiva has changed
- Introduce new instruments if necessary

ASSESSMENT AND TREATMENT OF MUCOSITIS

- Distinguish between generalized and local recurrence
- Analyze possible causes of reinfection
- Remove plaque around the implant using floss chosen in relation to the space between the peri-implant mucosa and the prosthesis
- Remove any deposits of calculus with carbon-fiber curettes and a sonic unit with a plastic tip

POLISHING OF IMPLANTS AND PROSTHESIS

- Remove any residual deposits and stains utilizing polishing paste with a low RDA

SCHEDULING OF THE NEXT RECALL
HEALTHY STATUS

- First year: recall every 3 or 4 months
- Following year: recall every 6 months

MUCOSITIS

- Recall after 3 months

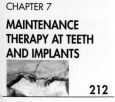
▶ REFERENCES

1. Adriaens PA, De Boever JA, Loeche WJ. Bacteria invasion in root cementum and radicular dentin of periodontally diseased teeth in humans. J Periodontol 1988;59:222–230.

2. Ainamo J, Bay I. Problems and proposals for recording gingivitis and plaque. Int Dent J 1975;25:229–235.

3. American Academy of Periodontology. Proceedings of the 3rd World Workshop in Clinical Periodontics, 23–27 July 1989, Princeton, NJ. Chicago: American Academy of Periodontology, 1989.

4. Axelsson P, Lindhe J. The effect of controlled oral hygiene procedures on caries and periodontal disease in adults. Results after 6 years. J Clin Periodontol 1981;8:239–248.

5. Axelsson P, Lindhe J. The significance of maintenance care in the treatment of periodontal disease. J Clin Periodontol 1981;8:281–294.

6. Badersten A, Nilvéus R, Egelberg J. Effect of nonsurgical periodontal therapy. I. Moderately advanced periodontitis. J Clin Periodontol 1981;8:57–72.

7. Badersten A, Nilvéus R, Egelberg J. Effect of nonsurgical periodontal therapy (VIII). Probing attachment changes related to clinical characteristics. J Clin Periodontol 1987;14:425–437.

8. Badersten A, Nilvéus R, Egelberg J. Scores of plaque, bleeding, suppuration and probing depths to predict probing attachment loss. J Clin Periodontol 1990;21:91–97.

9. Becker BE, Karp CL, Becker W, Berg LE. Personality differences and stressful life events. Differences between treated periodontal patients with and without maintenance. J Clin Periodontol 1988; 15:49–52.

10. Becker W, Becker BE, Berg LE. Periodontal treatment without maintenance. A retrospective study in 44 patients. J Periodontol 1984;55:505–509.

11. Berglundh T, Lindhe J, Ericsson I, Marinello CP, Liljenberg B. Soft tissue reactions to de novo plaque formation at implants and teeth. An experimental study in the dog. Clin Oral Implants Res 1992;3:1–8.

12. Berglundh T, Lindhe J, Ericsson I, Marinello CP, Liljenberg B, Thomsen P. The soft tissue barrier at implants and teeth. Clin Oral Implants Res 1991;2:81–90.

13. Bergström J, Blomlöf L. Tobacco smoking: A major risk factor associated with refractory periodontal disease [abstract 1530]. J Dent Res 1992;71(special issue):297.

14. Caton JG, Proye M, Polson A. Maintenance of healed periodontal pockets after a single episode of root planing. J Periodontol 1982;53:420–424.

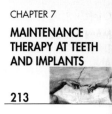
15. Checchi L, Pelliccioni GA, Gatto MR, Kelescian L. Patient compliance with maintenance therapy in an Italian periodontal practice. J Clin Periodontol 1994;21:309–312.

16. Claffey N, Nylund K, Kiger R, Garret S, Egelberg J. Diagnostic predictability of scores of plaque, bleeding, suppuration, and probing pocket depths for probing attachment loss. 3 1/2 years of observation following initial therapy. J Clin Periodontol 1990;17:108–114.

17. Demetriou N, Tsami-Pandi A, Parashis A. Compliance with supportive periodontal treatment in private periodontal practice. A 14-year retrospective study. J Periodontol 1995;66:145–149.

18. Dennison D, Lucye H, Suomi JD. Effects of dental health instruction on university students. J Am Dent Assoc 1974;89:1313–1317.

19. Elliot JR, Bowers GM, Clemmer BA, Rovelstad GH. Evaluation of an oral physiotherapy center in the reduction of bacterial plaque and peridontal disease. J Periodontol 1972;43:221–224.

20. Ericsson I, Berglundh T, Marinello CP, Liljenberg B, Lindhe J. Long-standing plaque and gingivitis at implants and teeth in the dog. Clin Oral Implants Res 1992;3:99–103.

21. Hill RW, Ramfjörd SP, Morrison EC, et al. Four types of periodontal treatment compared over two years. J Periodontol 1981;52:655–662.

22. Hirschfeld L., Wasserman B. A long-term survey of tooth loss in 600 treated periodontal patients. J Periodontol 1978;49:225–237.

23. Isidor F, Karring T. Long-term effect of surgical and non-surgical periodontal treatment. A 5-year clinical study. J Periodontal Res 1986;21:462–472.

24. Kerr NW. Treatment of chronic periodontitis. 45% failure rate after 5 years. Br Dent J 1981;50:222–224.

25. Knowles JW, Burgett F, Nissle RR, Shick RA, Morrison EC, Ramfjörd SP. Results of periodontal treatment related to pocket depth and attachment level. Eight years. J Periodontol 1979;50:225–233.

26. Lang NP, Adler R, Joss A, Nyman S. Absence of bleeding on probing. An indicator of periodontal stability. J Clin Periodontol 1990;17:714–721.

27. Lang NP, Joss A, Orsanic T, Gusberti FA, Siegrist BE. Bleeding on probing. A predictor for the progression of periodontal disease? J Clin Periodontol 1986;13:590–596.

28. Lang NP, Kiel R, Anderhalden K. Clinical and microbiological effects of subgingival restorations with overhanging or clinically perfect margins. J Clin Periodontol 1983;10:563–578.

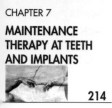
29. Lang NP, Nyman S, Senn C, Joss A. Bleeding on probing as it relates to probing pressure and gingival health. J Clin Periodontol 1991;18:257–261.

30. Lindhe J. Clinical Periodontology and Implant Dentistry, ed 3. Copenhagen: Munksgaard, 1997:chap 17, 27, 29.

31. Lindhe J, Berglundh T, Ericsson I, Liljenberg B, Marinello CP. Experimental breakdown of peri-implant and periodontal tissue. A study in the beagle dog. Clin Oral Implants Res 1992;3:9–16.

32. Lindhe J, Nyman S. The effect of plaque control and surgical pocket elimination on the establishment and maintenance of periodontal health. A longitudinal study of periodontal therapy in cases of advanced disease. J Clin Periodontol 1975;2:67–79.

33. Lindhe J, Nyman S. Long-term maintenance of patients treated for advanced periodontal disease. J Clin Periodontol 1984;11:504–514.

34. Lindhe J, Nyman S, Karring T. Scaling and root planing in shallow pockets. J Clin Periodontol 1982;9:415–418.

35. Lindhe J, Socransky SS, Nyman S, Haffajee A, Westfelt E. "Critical probing depths" in periodontal therapy. J Clin Periodontol 1982;9:323–336.

36. Listgarten MA, Lindhe J, Helldén L. Effect of tetracycline and/or scaling on human periodontal disease. Clinical, microbiological and histological observations. J Clin Periodontol 1978; 5:246–271.

37. Löe H, Ånerud Å, Boysen H, Morrison EC. Natural history of periodontal disease in man. Rapid, moderate and no loss of attachment in Sri Lankan laborers 14–46 years of age. J Clin Periodontol 1986;13:431–440.

38. Löe H, Ånerud Å, Boysen H, Smith M. The natural history of periodontal disease in man. The role of periodontal destruction before 40 years. J Periodontal Res 1978;49:607–620.

39. Loos B, Nylund K, Claffey N, Egelberg J. Clinical effects of root debridement in molar and non-molar teeth: A 2-year follow-up. J Clin Periodontol 1989;16:498–504.

40. Matarasso S, Quaremba G, Coraggio F, Vaia E, Cafiero C, Lang NP. Maintenance of implants: An in vitro study of titanium implant surface modifications subsequent to the application of different prophylaxis procedures. Clin Oral Implants Res 1996;7:64–72.

41. McFall WT. Tooth loss in 100 treated patients with periodontal disease in a long-term study. J Periodontol 1982;53:539–549.

42. Mendoza AR, Newcomb GM, Nixon KC. Compliance with supportive periodontal therapy. J Periodontol 1991;62:731–736.

43. Mombelli A, Nyman S, Brägger U, Wennström J, Lang NP. Clinical and microbiological changes associated with an altered subgingival environment induced by periodontal pocket reduction. J Clin Periodontol 1995;22:780–787.

44. Morrison EC, Lang NP, Löe H, Ramfjörd SP. Effects of repeated scaling and root planing and/or controlled oral hygiene on periodontal attachment level and pocket depth in beagle dogs. I. Clinical findings. J Periodontal Res 1979;14:428–437.

45. Mousquès T, Listgarten MA, Phillips RW. Effect of scaling and root planing on the composition of the human subgingival microbial flora. J Periodontal Res 1980;15:144–151.

46. Nordland P, Garrett S, Kiger R, Vanooteghem R, Hutchens LH, Egelberg J. The effect of plaque control and root debridement in molar teeth. J Clin Periodontol 1987;14:231–236.

47. Nyman S, Lindhe J. A longitudinal study of combined periodontal and prosthetic treatment of patients with advanced periodontal disease. J Periodontol 1979;50:163–169.

48. Nyman S, Lindhe J, Rosling B. Periodontal surgery in plaque-infected dentitions. J Clin Periodontol 1977;4:240–249.

49. Nyman S, Rosling B, Lindhe J. Effect of professional tooth cleaning on healing after periodontal surgery. J Clin Periodontol 1975;2:80–86.

50. Nyman S, Sarhed G, Ericsson I, Gottlow J, Karring T. Role of "diseased" root cementum in healing following treatment of periodontal disease. An experimental study in the dog. J Periodontal Res 1986;21:496–503.

51. Nyman S, Westfelt E, Sarhed G, Karring T. Role of "diseased" root cementum in healing following treatment of periodontal disease. A clinical study. J Clin Periodontol 1988;15:464–468.

52. O'Leary TJ, Drake RB, Naylor JE. The plaque control record. J Periodontol 1972;43:38.

53. Pihlström BL, McHugh RB, Oliphant TH, Ortiz-Campos C. Comparison of surgical and non-surgical treatment of periodontal disease. A review of current studies and additional results after 6 1/2 years. J Clin Periodontol 1983;10:524–541.

54. Ramfjörd SP. Maintenance care for treated periodontitis patients. J Clin Periodontol 1987;14:433–437.

55. Ramfjörd SP, Caffesse RG, Morrison EC, et al. Four modalities of periodontal treatment compared over 5 years. J Clin Periodontol 1987;14:445–452.

56. Ramfjörd SP, Morrison EC, Burgett FG, et al. Oral hygiene and maintenance of periodontal support. J Periodontol 1982;53:26–30.

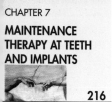
57. van Steenberghe D, Klinge B, Lindén U, Quirynen M, Herrmann I, Garpland C. Periodontal indices around natural titanium abutements: A longitudinal multicenter study. J Periodontol 1993;64:538–541.

58. Westfelt E, Bragd L, Socransky SS, Haffajee AD, Nyman S, Lindhe J. Improved periodontal conditions following therapy. J Clin Periodontol 1985;12:283–293.

59. Westfelt E, Nyman S, Socransky SS, Lindhe J. Significance of frequency of professional tooth cleaning for healing following periodontal surgery. J Clin Periodontol 1983;10:148–156.

60. Wilson TG. Compliance. A review of the literature with possible applications to periodontics. J Periodontol 1987;58:706–714.

61. Wilson TG, Glover ME, Malik AK, Schoen JA, Dorsett D. Tooth loss in maintenance patients in a private periodontal practice. J Periodontol 1987;58:231–235.

INDEX

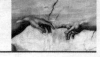

The image that appears on the cover and also accompanies all pages of the text was selected to confer a special significance to this book. In the scene of the creation of Adam, symbol of our renaissance, Michelangelo immortalizes the instant at which the first spark of life is kindled and passes from God's index finger to that of the first man on earth, and thereafter to the whole human race. Over millions of years, this vital force was transmitted, together with the human desire to gain knowledge and learn from the experience of others. The progress made by man and civilization, and the natural processes of evolution and selection, have determined the world of today. Not only great discoveries have helped to favor the evolution of our civilization, but also the small daily steps forward represented by the simple teachings handed down from parent to child and from teacher to student. This manual is an attempt to add a small drop to the never-ending flow of this transmission of experience, and if the reader benefits even in the slightest way from my endeavors, the book will have fulfilled its purpose.

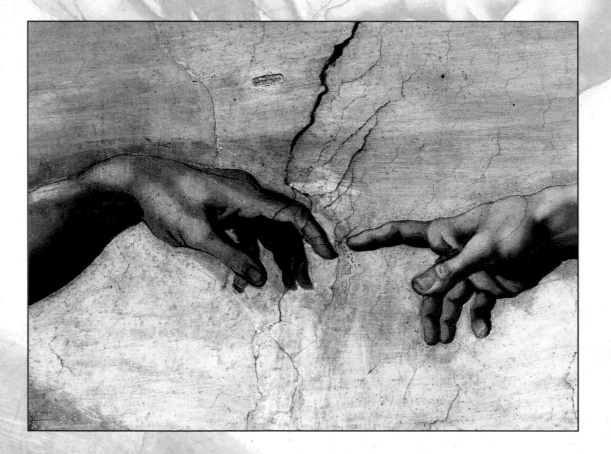

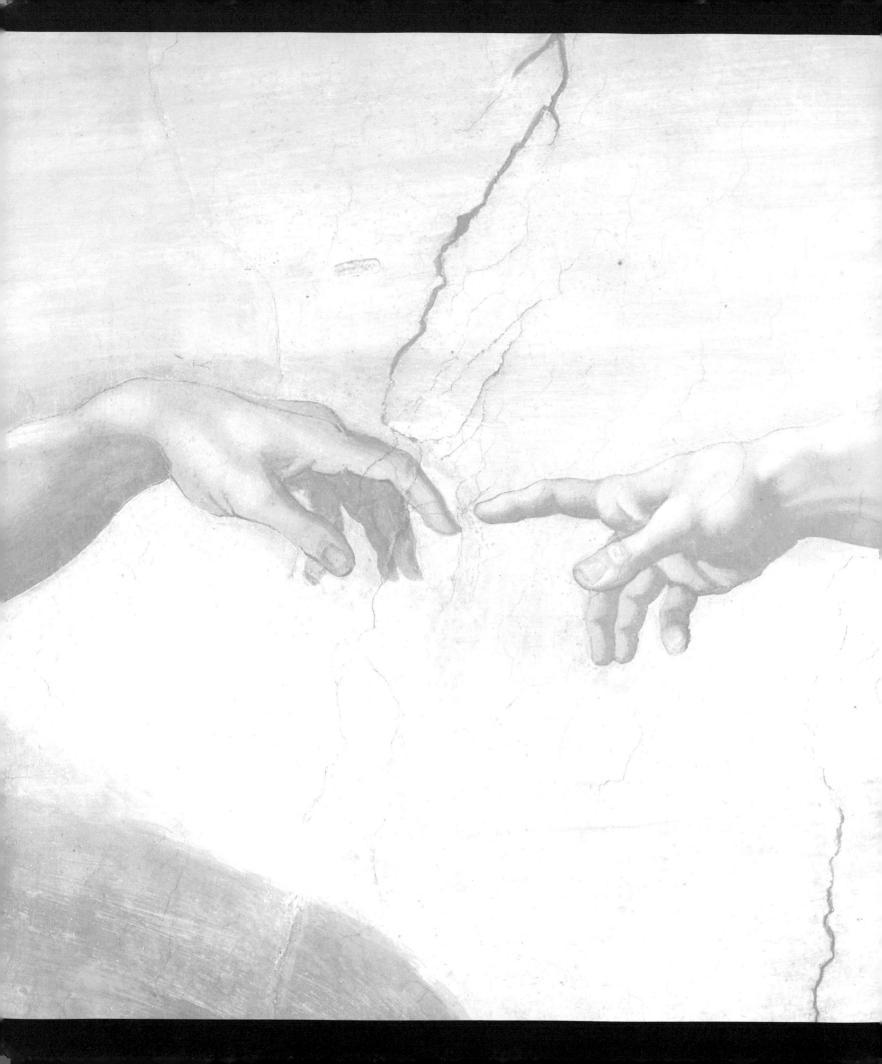

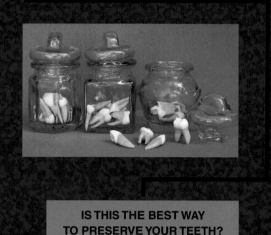

**IS THIS THE BEST WAY
TO PRESERVE YOUR TEETH?**

Each copy of *Experience Is the Best Teacher* contains one sample copy of the patient information handout entitled "Is This the Best Way to Preserve Your Teeth?" This 16-page handout explains in simple terms all of the fundamental aspects of periodontal disease, including its symptoms, etiology, progression, and treatment. Most importantly, the handout stresses the importance of patient compliance and cooperation.

The handout is useful as a visual guide, reference, and motivator, both in the office and in the patient's home. You can purchase additional copies of this informative handout to give to your patients. Each packet contains 25 handouts. Price: US $30, £ 25.

To order the patient handout, contact the Quintessence office in your area or send in the order form below.

▷ Quintessence Publishing Co, Ltd
Grafton Road, New Malden
Surrey, KT3 3AB, UK
Phone: 44 (0) 20 8949 6087
Fax: 44 (0) 20 8336 1484
Email: info@quintbook.co.uk

▷ Quintessence Publishing Co, Inc
551 Kimberly Drive
Carol Stream, IL 60188-1881, USA
Phone: (800) 621-0387
Fax: (630) 682-3288
Email: service@quintbook.com
Website: www.quintpub.com

ORDER FORM

Please send me____packets (containing 25 copies each) of "Is This the Best Way to Preserve Your Teeth?"

NAME_____

ADDRESS_____

CITY_____STATE_____ZIP_____

COUNTRY_____

PHONE_____FAX_____

❏ Charge to my credit card plus shipping & handling

❏ Visa   ❏ MC   ❏ AmEx   ❏ Discover

Card no._____ Exp._____

Signature_____

Prices subject to change without notice. All sales are final. Shipping and handling charges will be added to all orders.